HAND
REFLEXOLOGY
for Practitioners

by the same author

Principles of Reflexology
What it is, how it works, and what it can do for you: Revised Edition
Nicola Hall
ISBN 978 1 84819 137 2
eISBN 978 0 85701 108 4

of related interest

Pocket Handbook of Body Reflex Zones Illustrated in Color
Guo Changqing Guoyan and Zhaiwei Liu Naigang
ISBN 978 1 84819 119 8
eISBN 978 0 85701 095 7

Zero Balancing
Touching the Energy of Bone
John Hamwee
Foreword by Fritz Smith, MD FCCAc
Illustrations by Gina Michaels
ISBN 978 1 84819 234 8
eISBN 978 0 85701 182 4

Japanese Holistic Face Massage
Rosemary Patten
ISBN 978 1 84819 122 8
eISBN 978 0 85701 100 8

The Mystery of Pain
Douglas Nelson
ISBN 978 1 84819 152 5
eISBN 978 0 85701 116 9

The Compassionate Practitioner
How to Create a Successful and Rewarding Practice
Jane Wood
ISBN 978 1 84819 222 5
eISBN 978 0 85701 170 1

Getting Better at Getting People Better
Creating Successful Therapeutic Relationships
Noah Karrasch
ISBN 978 1 84819 239 3
eISBN 978 0 85701 186 2

'As a highly respected practitioner and advocate for complementary medicine, Nicola Hall is one of the most influential experts in the world of reflexology. Having benefited from her gentle but effective treatment of a long-standing sports injury, I can thoroughly recommend her deep knowledge and passion for her subject. These emerge in her vividly-written, thought-provoking book, which makes clear how hand reflexology, though less widely used than treatments of the feet, has a highly effective role to play in treating and alleviating a variety of conditions. Although aimed at the practitioner, the book is full of insights that will fascinate the general reader and help to strip away some of the myths and misapprehensions surrounding this ancient and accessible therapy.'

– Sally Jones, Journalist and Broadcaster

HAND
REFLEXOLOGY
for Practitioners

REFLEX AREAS, CONDITIONS AND TREATMENTS

NICOLA HALL
Foreword by Matthew Williams

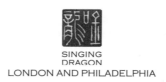

SINGING
DRAGON
LONDON AND PHILADELPHIA

Hand chart on page 188 is reproduced with kind permission from Lynne Booth.

First published in 2016
by Singing Dragon
an imprint of Jessica Kingsley Publishers
73 Collier Street
London N1 9BE, UK
and
400 Market Street, Suite 400
Philadelphia, PA 19106, USA

www.singingdragon.com

Library of Congress Cataloging in Publication Data
Hall, Nicola (Reflexologist), author.
 A practitioner's guide to hand reflexology / Nicola Hall ; foreword by Matthew Williams.
  p. ; cm.
 Includes bibliographical references and index.
 ISBN 978-1-84819-280-5 (alk. paper) -- ISBN 978-1-84819-247-8 (alk. paper)
 I. Title.
 [DNLM: 1. Massage--methods. 2. Hand. WB 537]
 RM721
 615.8'22--dc23
                    2015036380

British Library Cataloguing in Publication Data
A CIP catalogue record for this book is available from the British Library.

ISBN 978 1 84819 280 5
eISBN 978 0 85701 227 2

Printed and bound in Great Britain

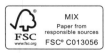

Contents

Foreword

The growth of complementary and alternative medicine, or integrated healthcare as it is now often called, has been driven over the past 30 years by patients who have wanted individual, patient-centred care that looks holistically at them as human beings rather than a group of conditions.

The demand for this type of care has come about because of the inability of conventional medicine to help with a range of common conditions, often long-term and chronic conditions where orthodox drugs and treatments have little success. Patients have increasingly sought non-invasive treatments with little or no side effects in preference to pharmaceutical drugs and surgical interventions.

Government and policymakers have been slow to catch up with the modern demands of patients, but groups such as the Parliamentary Group for Integrated Healthcare have driven the agenda centrally, whilst organisations around the UK, such as the British Reflexology Association, have worked to improve standards and professionalism among practitioners, provide patient choice and enable patients to access the kind of patient-centred care that modern healthcare demands.

I recall the Parliamentary Group for Integrated Healthcare hosting an exhibition at Westminster many years ago, and we decided that the therapy we would showcase was reflexology, because it was non-invasive, gentle and easy for Parliamentarians not familiar with complementary therapies to engage with. Reflexology was well received by all those who experienced it, which is not surprising because the philosophy behind reflexology epitomises why complementary therapies are so successful – it treats not just the symptoms, but the causes of the symptoms.

I have known Nicola Hall for almost 20 years. Since she trained in 1977 she has written eight or nine books on reflexology and is Director of the Bayly School of Reflexology, which was the first reflexology training school to be established in Great Britain in 1978. Nicola trained with the founder, the late Doreen Bayly, and is now regarded as a leading figure in the reflexology world and an important contributor to the development of complementary healthcare more widely. She previously had a clinic in London, is chairman of The British Reflexology Association and continues to be a valued member of the All-Party Parliamentary Group for Integrated Healthcare.

Nicola is well-respected throughout the field of integrated healthcare, far beyond the practice of reflexology. I have no doubts that with her vast knowledge, experience and professionalism, this book will prove to be a valuable publication for anyone wanting to learn about hand reflexology.

Matthew Williams
Manager, Parliamentary Group for Integrated Healthcare
Director, Integrated Healthcare Partnership
United Kingdom

Acknowledgements

I express special thanks to those who have contributed to this book by helping with the text on some of the different approaches to hand reflexology and hand treatments. These professionals include Philippe Mathon, Lynne Booth and Jong Baik, all of whom have made significant contributions to the practice of reflexology. Their details can be found in the Resources at the end of the book. I also give special thanks to Debbie Androlia for taking the photographs of a treatment session and to Maureen Androlia for acting as the client receiving treatment. Finally, I thank Nathalie Clarke of Pace Print and Design, Worcester UK, for her help in redesigning the hand chart on pages 33 and 44.

Preface

I was first introduced to reflexology in 1977 and was fortunate enough to be put in touch with the late Doreen Bayly with whom I trained and then assisted with her training courses. Myself and my colleague, Noelle Weyeneth, who runs a course for the Bayly School in Switzerland, are probably two of the few people still actively involved in reflexology who trained with Doreen Bayly, who is considered by many to have been the pioneer of reflexology in the UK and other parts of Europe.

There are many different approaches to reflexology treatment, and this book covers the approach that I follow and teach at the Bayly School, as well as explains the differences in approaches. There are also many different charts showing the positions of reflex areas in the feet and hands, but provided there is a rationale for the positioning of the reflex points, it would be incorrect to say which is right or which is wrong.

With the greater acceptance of complementary therapies since the time when I first trained, it is essential for all reflexology practitioners to be well qualified. The method of reflexology may seem a very simple one, but in order to practise professionally and to help others, a sound understanding of not just reflexology but also anatomy, physiology and pathology is required.

Although I have written a number of books on reflexology, this is the first to concentrate just on hand reflexology. The use of hand reflexology is probably underestimated, though there are some practitioners that I know of who *only* use hand reflexology, rather than foot reflexology. I recommend that all practitioners become more familiar with hand reflexology and more confident at giving hand reflexology treatments, as it has much to offer.

Reflexology has not yet received the respect that it deserves as a complementary therapy, but with integrated healthcare becoming more acceptable, it is hoped that as time passes, more and more people will have access to reflexology either through private practice or the health service in the UK. There are few people who experience reflexology treatment who do not benefit to some degree.

Chapter 1

General Introduction to Reflexology

When people think of reflexology they usually think of feet, and that it is a type of treatment given to the feet but for treating the body rather than treating problems involving the feet themselves. However, the widely accepted definition of reflexology (as described in the core curriculum for *Reflexology* published by the Reflexology Forum in the UK in 2006) is that reflexology is a form of complementary therapy involving treatment of reflex points and reflex areas found in the feet and the hands which relate to corresponding parts of the body. As well as foot and hand reflexology, more recently other approaches to reflexology have emerged such as ear reflexology, facial reflexology and scalp reflexology, but these approaches are probably more accurately described as forms of acupressure since they involve the meridians being worked on during acupuncture therapy. These microsystems certainly exist (and are referred to later in the book) and offer useful forms of treatment, but including the term 'reflexology' in the nomenclature is perhaps misleading.

Reflexology treatment to the hands is not as common as that to the feet, and many reflexology practitioners rarely use treatment to the hands even though most will have had an introduction to hand reflexology during their training. This book is a detailed guide to using hand reflexology and will be of interest to both reflexology practitioners wishing to offer this form of treatment and to those without formal training in reflexology but who might like to try some treatment on themselves. There are many instances when hand reflexology can be of use, and this book will hopefully enforce this view and encourage the use of this form of treatment more widely.

In the hands, as in the feet, there are reflex points and areas relating to all the different parts of the body, so it is possible to treat the whole body through the hands. Treatment to the areas is given using thumb or finger pressure to the precise reflex points and the technique involved is described in Chapter 5. There are a few instances when reflexology treatment might not be appropriate, but for the majority of cases, reflexology treatment may be very beneficial towards clearing symptoms or easing symptoms. Nearly everyone who has reflexology treatment finds that it is very relaxing, so it is helpful in reducing stress and tension, which are often causes or contributory factors to health problems.

Chapter 2

History and Theory
of Reflexology

Reflexology is an ancient form of complementary therapy, and the first pictorial evidence of a method such as reflexology being used is found in Egyptian tomb drawings. Furthermore, an ancient papyrus scene (dated 2500 BC) shows one man holding another man's foot and applying the thumb to a part of the foot in a manner as is used in reflexology treatment. The positions of the patients and that of the practitioners are different for the foot and hand treatments but neither are similar to those used in the modern-day practice of reflexology. The papyrus is from the tomb of Ankhmahor, a physician, and can be found at Saqqara in Egypt. The hieroglyphic above the scene shows one of the patients saying, 'Do not let it be painful' and with one of the practitioners replying, 'I do as you please'.

It is thought that reflexology or a similar method spread from Egypt to Greece, Arabia and then on to Europe through the Roman Empire. Evidence of the knowledge of therapies involving the application of pressure to the feet has also been traced back to India and Japan, with drawings showing mapping on the feet having been found in Japan (690 AD), Tibet, India and China. There is little evidence of these points on the hands, though.

It was also thought that the Incas used foot treatments, though there is no written record of this. Similarly, the American Indians, in particular the Cherokees, practised a form of reflexology, and it has been reported how this method was passed down through the generations. Whether or not hand reflexology was also used is not known.

Zone therapy (Dr William Fitzgerald)

The method of reflexology was brought to the attention of the Western world in the early 1900s initially through the work of Dr William Fitzgerald, an American ear, nose and throat specialist. Fitzgerald became very interested in various pressure therapies whilst studying in Europe and introduced a method which he called 'zone therapy' and of which he probably became aware whilst in Europe. A book on zone therapy by two European doctors, Dr Adamus and Dr A'tatis, had been published in 1582, and another book on zone therapy was published shortly after this by a Dr Ball. Based on zone therapy ideas, Dr Fitzgerald described how the body could be divided into ten longitudinal zones with each zone extending from the toes up the body to the brain and down the arms to the fingers. Each of the ten zones was of equal width at any point in the body and the zones were numbered according to which toe or finger they were in line with. There were five zones on the right side and five zones on the left side as follows:

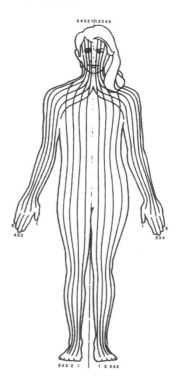

- Zone 1 extended from the big toe up the inner side of the leg, through the body up to the head and down the inner side of the arm to the thumb.

- Zone 2 extended from the second toe up the leg, through the body up to the head and down the arm to the second finger.

- Zone 3 extended from the third toe up the leg, through the body up to the head and down the arm to the third finger.

- Zone 4 extended from the fourth toe up the leg, through the body up to the head and down the arm to the fourth finger.

Longitudinal zones

- Zone 5 extended from the fifth (little) toe up the outer side of the leg, through the body up to the head and down the outer side of the arm to the fifth (little) finger.

The method of zone therapy involved applying pressure to a part of the body to influence the functioning of another part of the body situated in the same longitudinal zone but distant from the part of the body to where pressure was applied. By applying pressure to a zone, it was considered that any disturbance or energy block within that zone could be cleared and that with the correct flow of energy the body parts in that zone would function correctly. Fitzgerald would use various gadgets to apply the pressure and these included rubber bands (which would be wrapped around the fingers), clothes pegs (which were clipped to fingers or toes), metal combs (which would be pressed into the palm of the hand) and metal clips (which were placed on the

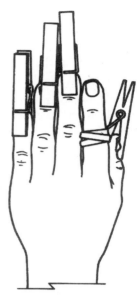

Gadgets used on hand

more fleshy parts of the body such as the abdomen). The gadgets would be used to apply a prolonged pressure with the patient being told only to release them when the area to which they were applied turned blue and was therefore being deprived of blood! This method was used mainly to relieve pain and also to act as an anaesthetic.

Fitzgerald's work, along with that of his colleagues Dr Edwin Bowers and Harry Bressler, did not receive much attention and did not really attract the interest of many others of Dr Fitzgerald's medical colleagues, but he did have successes and a number of devotees. In 1917 Fitzgerald and Bowers published a book called *Zone Therapy* (Fitzgerald and Bowers 1980). One physician who did believe in Fitzgerald's work was Dr Joe Shelby Riley, and together with his wife, Elizabeth, he used zone therapy in his practice for many years. His first book, *Zone Therapy Simplified*, was published in 1919 (Riley 2010). Riley also included work on the ear, and instead of gadgets for applying pressure (as Fitzgerald used), he developed a 'hooking' technique using the fingers.

Eunice Ingham

During the early 1930s, Eunice Ingham (1879–1974) worked with Dr Riley in Florida and it was Ingham who separated work on the reflexes of the feet from zone therapy in general. Ingham was the first person to describe the method of reflexology as it is widely known today, and it was she who first described the positions of reflex areas in the feet relating to the parts of the body and compiled a foot chart to show the positions of these reflex areas. The areas were apparently worked out by 'trial and error' with Ingham finding people with specific conditions that had been medically diagnosed as being present and then finding which areas of the feet were most sensitive to precise massage. From her research, she produced a foot chart which showed how the reflex areas of the feet formed a map of the body in the feet and she established her form of treatment named 'The Eunice Ingham Method of Compression Massage'. Ingham was also the first person to write on the subject of modern-day reflexology publishing her first book *Stories the Feet Can Tell* in 1938 followed by *Stories the Feet Have Told* in 1951 (Ingham and Byers 1992). Ingham was assisted in later years by her nephew, Dwight Byers, and his sister, Eusebia Messenger. There does not, however, appear to be evidence of Ingham compiling hand charts to show positions of reflex areas in the hands.

Doreen Bayly

One of the first reflexology hand charts produced was that of Doreen Bayly. Bayly introduced reflexology to Great Britain in the 1960s. She had been visiting her sister in America and through a friend of her sister was introduced to Eunice Ingham. She was fascinated by the method of reflexology and remained in America for a while to study with Ingham. She then returned to England to try to establish the method outside of America, and although there was not a great interest in the various forms of complementary medicine in the 1960s, Bayly was determined to introduce the method of reflexology to as many people as possible in order that they could experience its wonderful effects. She set up a reflexology practice in London and would treat a number of people, and she also started to run small training classes to teach others to practise the method. In those early days, certification for the courses came from Eunice Ingham in America. Over the years, the interest in reflexology grew with more and more people keen to try treatment and to train in the method. Doreen Bayly lectured not only in Great Britain but also in Europe, and following the death of Eunice Ingham she started The Bayly School of Reflexology which was the first reflexology training school to be established in Great Britain. Bayly's book, *Reflexology Today*, published in 1978, was the first text on the subject to be published in Europe and did include a basic hand chart to show reflex areas that could be worked on in the hands (Bayly 1988).

Mildred Carter

One of the early practitioners of hand reflexology was Mildred Carter, an American. Carter was self-taught from reading a book on reflexology that she had been given by a relative. She began practising the method to support her three children, having been widowed and being without a source of income. Her practice developed quickly, and in 1954 she attended a training course with Eunice Ingham to obtain a certificate. However, the practice of reflexology in her state was not lawful and she met with much opposition to her work, particularly when she had her first book on reflexology published in 1968. She gave up her practice because of this but still continued to work on family and friends and to write more books. Her book, *Hand Reflexology: Key to Perfect Health*, was published in 1975 and was one of the first books on hand reflexology (Carter 1975). Her approach to treatment was very much based on zone therapy principles and she used different gadgets to apply pressure to the reflex areas in the hands and also encouraged self-treatment.

Transverse zones

Another important contribution to the theory of reflexology was made by a German practitioner, Hanne Marquardt. It was Marquardt who first described the transverse zones of reflexology which were helpful in determining the position of the reflex areas. The transverse zones were explained as relating to the level of the shoulder girdle, the level of the waist and the level of the pelvic floor. These transverse zones (or lines) could be described in relation to the bones of the feet as follows:

- The first zone is at the base of the phalanges where they meet the metatarsals, and this relates to the level of the shoulder girdle.

- The second zone is at the base of the metatarsals where they meet the tarsals, and this relates to the level of the waist.

- The third zone cuts across the talus on the sole of the foot and the lower end of the tibia (the larger bone of the lower leg) on the upper part of the foot, and is equivalent to an imaginary line between the two ankle bones (malleoli). This relates to the level of the pelvic floor.

An additional transverse zone useful to the reflexologist is the level of the diaphragm, and in the foot this is described as being an area across the metatarsals below the head of the first metatarsal (just below the ball of the foot).

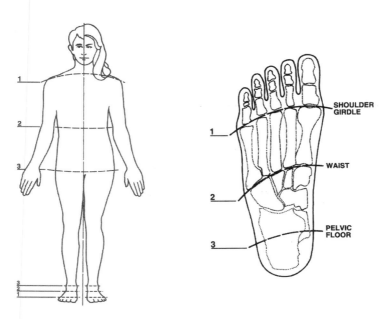

Transverse zones in the body and feet

These transverse zones do not relate so precisely to the joints between the bones in the hands, so they are less accurately located but they are still useful in determining the position of reflex areas.

In the hands, the level of the shoulder girdle is where the phalanges meet the metacarpals, and the level of the diaphragm is across the palm of the hand extending from about the level of the 'crease' mark found approximately 1 cm from the base of the little finger. The level of the waist is halfway down the palm of the hand extending to the area halfway down from the base of the thumb to the wrist (not equivalent to where the metacarpals meet the carpals). This zone can be more difficult to locate since it depends on the shape of the hand and the depth of the angle of the thumb. The level of the pelvic floor is across the carpal bones above the wrist.

The longitudinal and transverse zones of reflexology enable the location of reflex areas to be established. Since the longitudinal zones extend throughout the body and end in the hands and feet, whichever longitudinal zone or zones of the body an organ is situated in, there will be a corresponding reflex area in the same longitudinal zone or zones of the hands and feet. The transverse zones divide the areas up further so that parts of the body found above the level of the shoulder girdle are represented by reflex areas found above the shoulder girdle in the hands and feet; parts of the body found between the shoulder girdle and diaphragm level are represented by reflex areas found between the shoulder girdle and diaphragm level in the hands and feet; parts of the body found between the diaphragm and the waist are represented by reflex areas found between the levels of the diaphragm and the waist in the hands and feet; parts of the body found between the waist and the pelvic floor are represented by reflex areas found between the levels of the waist and the pelvic floor in the hands and feet; parts of the body found below the level of the pelvic floor are represented by reflex areas found below the level of the pelvic floor in the hands and feet.

There is therefore a grid-like pattern produced by the longitudinal and transverse zones to divide the hands and feet into areas corresponding to body areas and which helps to identify reflex areas for all parts of the body. The exact positions of these reflex areas are discussed in Chapter 4.

Zone-related areas

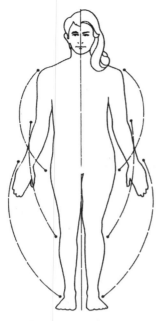

Zone-related areas

Having described the ten longitudinal zones of the body, Dr Fitzgerald also described the existence of additional areas known as zone-related areas (sometimes referred to as cross-reflexes or referral areas), which can be incorporated into reflexology treatment. The term 'zone-related areas' is preferable to 'cross-reflexes' as the latter term is perhaps a bit misleading since nothing actually crosses over. With the ten longitudinal zones present in both the arms and legs, the arm and the leg on the same side of the body are said to be zone-related. There exists a more precise link between the shoulder and the hip, the elbow and the knee, the hand and the foot, and the fingers and the toes on the same side. Similarly, the areas in between the joints of the limbs would be 'zone-related' with the upper arm relating to the upper leg and the forearm (lower arm) relating to the lower leg. Therefore, in addition to the reflexology treatment to the hands, the zone-related areas can be worked on directly (or through the corresponding reflex area) for specific problems. For example, massage to the right elbow might help a problem in the right knee or massage to the left wrist for a problem in the left ankle. These zone-related areas can sometimes be of great help, so they are always worth remembering.

The theories put forward by Dr William Fitzgerald, Eunice Ingham and Hanne Marquardt form the basis of reflexology treatment whether involving the feet or the hands. To date, there is no firm scientific evidence to support the existence of all of the reflex areas in the feet or the hands, but those working with the method can testify to the effectiveness of treatment and how tender areas in the feet or hands directly relate to problems existing in the body.

Chapter 3

Anatomy of the Hand

Since the hands are to be worked on in hand reflexology, it is useful to have an understanding of the basic anatomy of the hand, which is quite detailed. Although similar in many ways to the feet, as humans have evolved from being four-footed to two-footed, the hands have evolved to perform more precise movements. In the true anatomical position, the body is viewed facing forwards with the palms of the hands facing forwards. Therefore, the thumb side would be accurately described as the lateral (outer) side of the hand and the little-finger side as the medial (inner) side of the hand. This is the reverse of the reflexology position involving the longitudinal zones when the body would be viewed with the palms of the hands facing backwards. Some additional anatomical terminology involving hands are the words pronation, meaning palm turned downwards, and supination, meaning palm turned upwards.

The hands are designed to provide the body with support and flexibility to enable objects to be manipulated in a variety of ways. With the arrangement of the bones in the hand supported by the many muscles from the forearm that manipulate these bones, there is the ability to carry out a very wide range of movements with great precision – holding on to objects to support the body, picking up small items, unscrewing jars, playing the piano and so forth.

Bones of the hands

The bones of the hand are similar to those found in the feet, but there are 27 bones in the hands compared with 26 bones in the feet. In each hand there are 14 phalanges, 5 metacarpal bones and 8 carpal bones.

The phalanges are the bones of the fingers, with each finger having 3 phalanges (a distal, intermediate and proximal phalanx), except for the thumb which has just 2 phalanges (no intermediate phalanx). The joints between the phalanges are hinge joints. The proximal phalanges articulate with the metacarpal bones. The fingers are often referred to by name rather than number with the thumb being the first finger, the second finger being termed the index finger, the third finger being the long finger, the fourth finger being the ring finger and the fifth finger being the small or little finger.

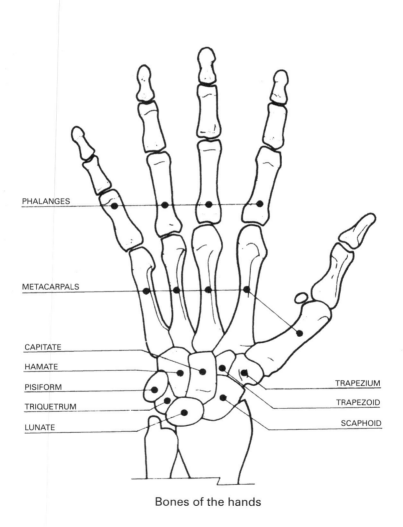

PHALANGES

METACARPALS

CAPITATE

HAMATE

PISIFORM

TRIQUETRUM

LUNATE

TRAPEZIUM

TRAPEZOID

SCAPHOID

Bones of the hands

The 5 metacarpal bones are long, thin bones with one in line with each finger, and these are numbered according to which finger they are in line with, that is, the first being in line with the thumb and the fifth being in line with the little finger. The metacarpal bones then articulate with the carpal bones.

The 8 carpal bones are arranged in two rows with 4 bones in each row. The bones of the distal row, which articulate with the metacarpal bones are, from the lateral (thumb) side, the trapezium, the trapezoid, the capitate and the hamate; the bones of the proximal row, from the lateral (thumb) side, are the scaphoid, the lunate, the triquetrum and the pisiform. The bones of the proximal row articulate with the bones of the forearm, radius (lateral side) and ulna (medial side), to form the wrist joint. There is very limited movement between the individual carpal bones, and there is restricted movement of the wrist joint, which is the most complex joint in the body. The wrist joint is a condyloid joint and is formed between the distal end of the radius and the proximal ends of the scaphoid, lunate and triquetral bones.

The thumb joint is particularly significant in being a highly mobile joint necessary to assist in the movements that the hand can perform. This mobility is due to the design of the joint between the first metacarpal bone and the trapezium bone and its many associated muscles. These hand bones are fitted closely together and held in position by ligaments. There are synovial joints between the carpal bones, between the carpals and metacarpals, between the metacarpals and proximal phalanges and between the phalanges.

Tendons of the muscles of the forearm cross the wrist and are held close to the bones of the hand by strong fibrous bands. There are also many small muscles within the hand.

Muscles of the hands

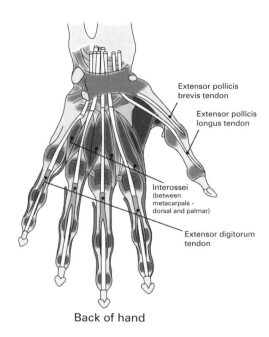

- Extensor pollicis brevis tendon
- Extensor pollicis longus tendon
- Interossei (between metacarpals - dorsal and palmar)
- Extensor digitorum tendon

Back of hand

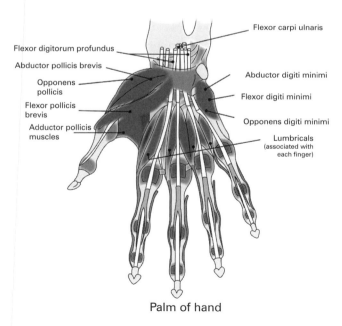

- Flexor digitorum profundus
- Abductor pollicis brevis
- Opponens pollicis
- Flexor pollicis brevis
- Adductor pollicis muscles
- Flexor carpi ulnaris
- Abductor digiti minimi
- Flexor digiti minimi
- Opponens digiti minimi
- Lumbricals (associated with each finger)

Palm of hand

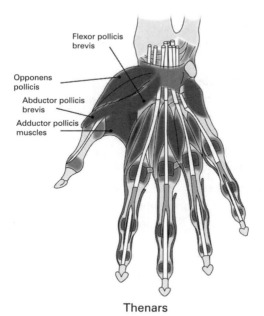

Flexor pollicis brevis

Opponens pollicis

Abductor pollicis brevis

Adductor pollicis muscles

Thenars

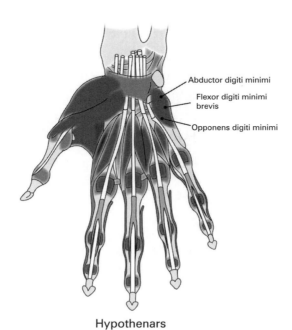

Abductor digiti minimi

Flexor digiti minimi brevis

Opponens digiti minimi

Hypothenars

The muscles of the hands are divided into intrinsic and extrinsic groups. The intrinsic muscles are found within the hand itself and the extrinsic muscles are found in the forearm and insert into the bones of the hand by long tendons. Muscles of the forearm flex and extend the phalanges of the hands by pulling on long tendons that run through the wrist and hand.

The intrinsic muscles can be divided into four groups – the thenar, hypothenar, lumbrical and interossei muscles. The thenar group is made up of the abductor pollicis brevis, flexor pollicis brevis, opponens pollicis and adductor pollicis muscles. All these muscles are innervated by the median nerve, except for the adductor pollicis and deep head of the flexor pollicis brevis.

Abductor pollicis brevis abducts the thumb; flexor pollicis brevis flexes and adducts the thumb; opponens pollicis draws the thumb across the palm to meet the little finger; and adductor pollicis adducts the thumb.

The extrinsic muscles include both flexors and extensors. All of the extrinsic extensor muscles are innervated by the radial nerve and this includes three wrist extensors and most of the thumb and finger extensors. The extrinsic flexor muscles are innervated by the median nerve, except for the flexor carpi ulnaris and flexor digitorum profundus to the small and ring fingers, which are innervated by the ulnar nerve. Therefore, in more simple terms, the muscles of the hand can be subdivided into three groups:

- those of the thumb which occupy the radial side and produce the thenar eminence

- those of the little finger which occupy the ulnar side and give rise to the hypothenar eminence

- those in the middle of the palm and between the metacarpal bones.

Nerves of the hands

The hand is supplied by three nerves – median, ulnar and radial – each of which has motor and sensory components.

The median nerve innervates the muscles involved in the fine precision and pinch function of the hand. This nerve innervates muscles of the anterior forearm, some of the muscles of the palm of the hand and the skin of the lateral palm and fingers. It enters the hand through the carpal tunnel and the sensory branch goes to the thumb, index finger, long finger and half of the ring finger; the motor branch goes to the thenar muscles of the thumb (abductor pollicis brevis, flexor pollicis brevis, opponens pollicis).

The ulnar nerve innervates the muscles involved in the power-grasping function of the hand. This nerve innervates the anteromedial muscles of the forearm, most of the muscles of the palm of the hand and the skin or the medial hand and fingers. It enters the hand through Guyon's canal and the sensory branch goes to the little finger and half of the ring finger. The motor branch goes to adductor pollicis and the hypothenar muscles (abductor digiti minimi, flexor digiti minimi brevis, opponens digiti minimi).

The radial nerve innervates the wrist extensors that control the position of the hand and stabilises it. This nerve innervates the muscles and skin of the posterior arm and forearm, the skin of the lateral hand and some fingers. It runs along the thumb-side edge of the forearm and gives sensation to the back of the hand from the thumb to the main knuckle of the back surface of the ring and middle fingers.

Skin of the hands

The skin covering the palm of the hand is different from that on the dorsum (back) of the hand. On the dorsum the skin is thin and pliable and somewhat loosely attached. The skin of the palmar surface is thicker and less pliable than that of the dorsum, and this allows greater stability of the skin to enable the hands to grasp objects. The skin of the palmar surface also contains numerous sensory nerve organs which are essential for the normal function of the hands.

Nails

Nails are a special type of cell that fills with hard keratin and grows over the epidermis of the skin at the ends of the fingers to act as a protective layer. The visible part of the nail is the nail body and the actively growing part of the nail is the white crescent-shaped lunula at the base of the nail. The nail root is the non-visible part below the lunula hidden by the cuticle. The nail bed is a layer of epithelium under the nail and it appears pink through the translucent nail body due to the presence of the many underlying blood capillaries. (If there is a drop in the level of oxygen in the blood, cyanosis develops and the nail bed will turn blue.)

Fingernails grow about 0.1 mm per day and grow three to four times faster than toenails. Generally, the longer the digit, the faster the nail grows, and it would take about six months for a fingernail to grow out. The nails tend to grow faster on the dominant hand and they grow faster in the summer and during pregnancy.

From the above description it is clear that in the small areas of the hands there are complex structures, and it is useful to be aware of this hand construction as the reflexologist is going to be working on these areas.

Chapter 4

Reflex Areas of the Hands

It has already been stated that there are areas in the hands that relate to all of the parts of the body, and both the palms of the hands and the backs of the hands contain these reflex areas. The reflex areas are arranged in such a manner that a map of the body can be found in the hands, though this body map is somewhat compressed compared with that formed in the feet, due to the smaller size of the hands. The right hand corresponds to the right side of the body and the left hand corresponds to the left side of the body, so parts of the body found on the right side are found in the right hand and parts of the body found on the left side are found in the left hand. For parts of the body that are found on both sides of the body these are represented in both hands (e.g. the right eye in the right hand and the left eye in the left hand). For parts of the body found on just one side of the body these are represented in the corresponding hand (e.g. the gall bladder, which is on the right side of the body, is represented in just the right hand, and the spleen, which is on the left side of the body, is represented in just the left hand).

When treating a particular reflex area, it refers to treating everything in that area, so this includes not only the actual organs or glands in a particular zone of the body but also the blood supply to the area, the nerve supply to the area, the muscles of the area and the skin covering the area. Thus, to treat the skin of a particular part, the corresponding reflex area would need to be worked (e.g. to treat the face, the facial reflex area would need to be worked).

For those familiar with foot reflexology and the position of reflex areas found in the feet, for hand reflexology the palm of the hand is equivalent to the sole of the foot, and the back of the hand is equivalent to the top of the foot. Those reflex areas which are found on the sole of the foot are also found in the palm of the hand, and those reflex areas found on the top of the foot are also found on the back of the hand.

In the foot there are reflex areas found on the medial border along the big-toe side of the foot, and these areas are found along the thumb-side edge of the hand (zone 1). The reflex areas found on the lateral border of foot are found along the little-finger side of the hand and also on the back of the hand (zone 5), since the hand does not have the same depth to the sides as is present in the foot.

With an understanding of where all the different parts are situated in the body in terms of the longitudinal and transverse zones, reflex areas can be identified in the similar zones of the hands. The explanations below examine the individual reflex areas to the main parts of the body with a short description of the part of the body to include where it is in the body and what it does, and then a description of the position of the reflex area(s) to this part.

Positions of the reflex areas of the hands

Palms of the hands

The majority of the parts of the body are represented in the palms of the hands, with those parts found on the right side of the body represented in the right hand and those parts found on the left side of the body represented in the left hand. In relation to the transverse zones of reflexology (described previously), the positioning of the reflex areas is as listed below.

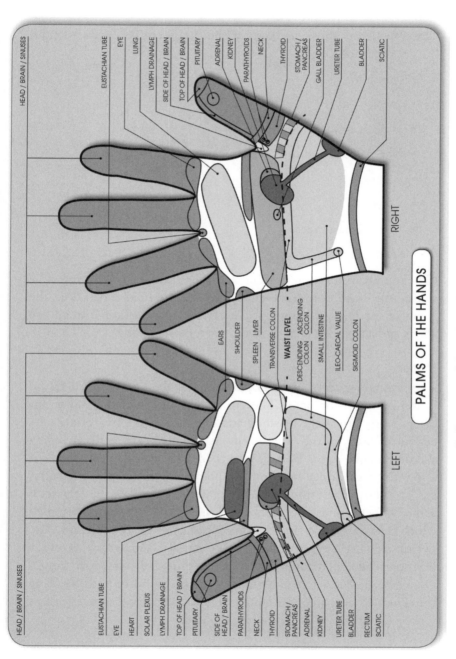

HEAD / BRAIN / SINUSES

EUSTACHIAN TUBE
EYE
HEART
SOLAR PLEXUS
LYMPH DRAINAGE
TOP OF HEAD / BRAIN
PITUITARY
SIDE OF HEAD / BRAIN
PARATHYROIDS
NECK
THYROID
STOMACH / PANCREAS
ADRENAL
KIDNEY
URETER TUBE
BLADDER
RECTUM
SCIATIC

LEFT

EARS
SHOULDER
SPLEEN
LIVER
TRANSVERSE COLON
WAIST LEVEL
DESCENDING COLON
ASCENDING COLON
SMALL INTESTINE
ILEO-CAECAL VALVE
SIGMOID COLON

HEAD / BRAIN / SINUSES

EUSTACHIAN TUBE
EYE
LUNG
LYMPH DRAINAGE
SIDE OF HEAD / BRAIN
TOP OF HEAD / BRAIN
PITUITARY
ADRENAL
KIDNEY
PARATHYROIDS
NECK
THYROID
STOMACH / PANCREAS
GALL BLADDER
URETER TUBE
BLADDER
SCIATIC

RIGHT

PALMS OF THE HANDS

Reflex areas of the palms of the hands

The reflex areas above the level of the shoulder girdle and over the fingers are as follows:

- pituitary
- neck
- side of head and side of brain
- top of head and top of brain
- sinuses
- eyes
- Eustachian tubes
- ears.

(The thumb, in addition to being zone 1, can also be considered to be sub-divided further to represent all five longitudinal zones; thus, the zones of the head and brain are represented in the thumb in all five zones and also in the fingers in the appropriate zone.)

Pituitary

The pituitary gland is a small gland, about the size of a pea, found in the centre of the brain. The pituitary is a hormonal gland and is often referred to as the master gland of the body since it controls the actions of many of the other hormonal glands in the body including the thyroid gland, the adrenal glands and the reproductive glands. It also influences kidney function and body growth. The hypothalamus lies just above the pituitary in the brain and controls the release of some of the pituitary hormones and itself produces some hormones which then pass to the pituitary for release into the bloodstream. Also positioned close to the pituitary is the pineal gland, which secretes a hormone called melatonin that influences the daily bodily rhythms.

The reflex area to the pituitary gland is found in both hands in the centre of the pad of the thumb. This also relates to the reflex area for the hypothalamus and the pineal gland.

Neck

The neck connects the head to the body, and in the back of the neck are various muscles which support the head to keep it upright.

The reflex area to the neck (back of neck) is found in both hands at the base of the thumb just above where it joins the palm.

Side of head and side of brain

The side of the head and the side of the brain refers to the outer side of the head and the brain as well as the side of the skull.

The reflex areas to the side of the head and the side of the brain are found in both hands up the side of the thumb (the side adjacent to the second finger).

Top of head and top of brain

The top of the head and the top of the brain refers to the upper parts of both the head and the brain as well as the top of the skull.

The reflex areas to the top of the head and the top of the brain are found in both hands across the top of the thumb.

Sinuses

The sinuses are air-filled cavities found in the skull behind the eyebrows, above and to the sides of the nose and below the eyes in the frontal, sphenoidal, ethmoidal and maxillary bones of the skull. They help reduce the weight of the head to allow it to rest on the spine. They link with the nose and are lined by cells which produce mucus.

The reflex areas to the sinuses are found in both hands up the palm side and sides of the second, third, fourth and fifth fingers.

Eyes

The eyes are the organs for sight and are situated within the orbital cavities in the front of the skull. Light rays pass through the lens of the eye to the back of the eye from where messages are sent by nerves to the regions of the brain responsible for vision.

The reflex areas to the eyes are found in both hands just below where the second and third fingers join the palm of the hand and slightly up the fingers.

Eustachian tubes

The Eustachian tubes connect the middle ear to the throat and are responsible for maintaining equal pressure on either side of the ear drum which is necessary for correct hearing.

The reflex areas to the Eustachian tubes are found in both hands in the palm just below the web between the third and fourth fingers.

Ears

The ears are the organs of hearing and also are important for balance. The outer ear leads down to the ear drum, and in the middle ear there are three small bones which are involved in the hearing process. The inner ear contains the receptors for hearing and for balance, and nerves from these areas pass to the regions of the brain responsible for hearing and balance.

The reflex areas to the ears are found in both hands just below where the fourth and fifth fingers join the palm of the hand.

REFLEX AREAS BETWEEN THE LEVELS OF THE SHOULDER GIRDLE AND THE DIAPHRAGM

The reflex areas between the levels of the shoulder girdle and the diaphragm are as follows:

- shoulders
- thyroid
- parathyroids
- lungs
- heart (left foot only)
- thymus.

Shoulders

The shoulder joint is where the arm attaches to the shoulder girdle of the upper body. This is a ball-and-socket joint with the head of the humerus (the bone of the upper arm) sitting in a socket on the outer side of the shoulder girdle.

The reflex areas to the shoulders are found just below the base of the little finger on the palm of the hand and also in a similar area on the back of the hand.

Thyroid and parathyroids

The thyroid gland is found in the front of the lower part of the neck. It produces hormones including thyroxine, which influences the metabolic rate in the body, and calcitonin, which influences the calcium levels in the blood.

The parathyroids are four small glands situated in the back of the thyroid gland and they produce a hormone, parathyroid hormone, which influences the level of calcium in the blood, working in an opposite way to the hormone from the thyroid.

The reflex areas to the thyroid are found in both hands in an area just below where the thumb joins the palm of the hand.

The reflex areas to the parathyroids are found in both hands on the outer margins (zone 2 side) of the thyroid area just below where the thumb joins the palm of the hand with an upper and lower reflex on each hand.

Lungs

The lungs are situated in the thoracic cavity (chest region) of the body and are responsible for breathing. The air breathed in takes oxygen into the body and the air breathed out contains carbon dioxide (a waste material). The lungs are cone shaped and can be described as having a tree-like structure with the main trunk of the tree, the trachea (windpipe), dividing into two main branches, the bronchi, which then divide into smaller branches called bronchioles, which occupy the lungs. The exchange of gases takes place through small air sacs at the end of the branches called alveoli. The membranes surrounding each lung are called the pleura, and the lungs are further protected by the ribs.

The reflex areas to the lungs are found in both hands in zones 2–5 in the palm of the hand below shoulder girdle level and above diaphragm level. These areas also relate to the areas for the ribs. The reflex areas for the bronchi extend across from zone 1 into the lung area in zone 2. (These reflex areas are not labelled in the diagram on page 34.)

Heart

The heart is situated in the chest region nearly centrally just above the diaphragm but with one-third to the right side and two-thirds to the left side. It is about the size of a clenched fist and can be divided into four chambers with an upper and a lower chamber, an atrium and a ventricle, respectively, on each side of the heart. Blood is pumped round the body by the heart and, once oxygenated, leaves the left side of the heart via the aorta, and the deoxygenated blood returns to the right side of the heart via veins (the inferior and superior vena cavae).

The reflex area to the heart is found in the palms of just the left hand mainly in zones 2 and 3 just above diaphragm level.

Thymus

The thymus is situated centrally in the upper part of the chest region between the lungs, and behind the sternum above the heart. It is largest at puberty but then reduces in size in adulthood. It is part of the lymphatic system and aids the development of the lymphocytes, cells able to respond to antigens in the body.

The reflex to the thymus is found in the palms of both hands in zone 1 just below the level of the shoulder girdle. (This reflex area is not labelled in the diagram on page 34.)

REFLEX AREAS BETWEEN DIAPHRAGM LEVEL AND WAIST LEVEL

The reflex areas between diaphragm level and waist level are as follows:

- solar plexus
- liver (right hand only)
- gall bladder (right hand only)
- spleen (left hand only)
- stomach
- pancreas.

Solar plexus

The solar plexus is a network of nerves situated just behind the diaphragm which gives off many nerve branches to supply parts in the abdomen.

The reflex areas to the solar plexus are found in the palms of both hands in zones 2 and 3 just below diaphragm level.

Liver

The liver is situated on the right side of the body below the diaphragm and has a triangular shape with its narrower lower margin ending just above waist level. It is a large organ and performs a large number of functions including the metabolism of food substances (it can make certain proteins and store glucose as an energy reserve), the manufacture of bile, the breakdown of alcohol, the storage of some vitamins and the detoxifying of substances that might be toxic to the body.

The reflex area to the liver is found in the palm of just the right hand in all five zones just below diaphragm level and tapering off to just zones 3–5 just above waist level.

Gall bladder

The gall bladder is attached to the lower margin of the liver, so it is found just above waist level on the right side of the body. The gall bladder stores the bile made in the liver and releases this into the small intestine when fats are eaten and aids in the digestion of the fats.

The reflex area to the gall bladder is found in the palm of just the right hand in zone 3 just above waist level.

Spleen

The spleen is found above the waist on the outer part of the left side of the body. It is important for breaking down old red blood cells and for activating new white blood cells, which play an important part in the body's defence system.

The reflex area to the spleen is found in the palm of just the left hand in zones 4 and 5 between the diaphragm and the waist.

Stomach

The stomach is found in the upper abdomen mainly on the left side but reaching slightly across to the right side. It is part of the digestive system and the food that is eaten passes down from the mouth to the throat and then into the oesophagus before reaching the stomach, where it is stored for a few hours and mixed with gastric juices, which begins the digestive process.

The reflex areas to the stomach are found in the palms of both hands in the area between the diaphragm and the waist in zones 1–3 on the left hand and the lower part of this area in zone 1 on the right hand. The reflex areas to the oesophagus extend from the throat area down the lateral border of zone 1 to lead into the stomach areas. (These reflex areas are not labelled in the diagram on page 34.)

Pancreas

The pancreas is situated fairly centrally in the body just above waist level and is overlapped by the stomach. The pancreas plays an important part in digestion by producing enzymes which travel down the pancreatic duct to the small intestine to help digest proteins, carbohydrates and fats. The pancreas also produces hormones, including insulin, which act to adjust the blood sugar levels.

The reflex areas to the pancreas are found in the palms of both hands in the lower half of the area between the diaphragm and the waist in zones 1–3 on the left hand and zone 1 on the right hand. (They are overlapped in much of this area by the reflex areas to the stomach.)

REFLEX AREAS BELOW WAIST LEVEL

The reflex areas below waist level are as follows:

- small intestine
- large intestine (ileo-caecal valve, ascending colon, transverse colon: right hand only; transverse colon, descending colon, sigmoid colon, rectum: left hand only)
- bladder
- ureter tubes
- kidneys
- adrenal glands
- sciatic nerves

Small intestine

The small intestine connects the stomach to the large intestine. It begins with a C-shaped area called the duodenum which then leads into tubing (the jejunum and the ileum), which lies folded back on itself within the abdomen. The main function of the small intestine is to break down the food that reaches it from the stomach into smaller particles, which can be absorbed through the walls of the small intestine (through special areas called villi) into the bloodstream.

The reflex areas to the small intestine are found in the palms of both hands in the area below waist level down to just above the wrist in zones 1–4.

Large intestine

The large intestine is a wide tube extending from the small intestine to the exterior and starts on the lower right side of the abdomen with the ileo-caecal valve (between the ileum of the small intestine and the caecum of the large intestine). The appendix is situated just off the caecum. The large intestine then passes up to waist level as the ascending colon and then stretches across waist level as the transverse colon. On the outer left side of the body is heads downwards as the descending colon before bending back towards the centre as the sigmoid colon. The sigmoid colon leads into the rectum which in turn leads into the anus. The main function of the large intestine is to eliminate (in the form of faeces) the undigested food that reaches it from the small intestine. As the undigested food travels through the large intestine, water is reabsorbed back into the body.

The reflex areas to the large intestine are found in the palms of both hands starting with the reflex area to the ileo-caecal valve in the right hand in zones 4 and 5 just above the wrist (this is also the area for the appendix) with the reflex area to the ascending colon extending upwards from this point to waist level. At waist level, the reflex area to the transverse colon starts in zones 4 and 5 and travels across all the zones in the right hand and across the left hand to zones 4 and 5. The reflex area to the descending colon travels down from waist level in zones 4 and 5 to just above the wrist, and then the reflex area to the sigmoid colon travels back to the centre across all the zones, finishing in zone 1 with the reflex area to the rectum and anus. (The reflex areas are described as being in zones 4 and 5 since they occupy a part of, but not the whole of, these zones.)

Bladder

The bladder is found centrally positioned in the pelvis and stores the urine produced by the kidneys until it is convenient to expel this from the body.

The reflex areas to the bladder are found in the palms of both hands in zone 1 just above the wrist and may also extend to a similar area just on the backs of the hands.

Ureter tubes

The two ureter tubes extend one on each side from the kidneys at waist level down to the bladder in the pelvic cavity. They are responsible for transporting the urine made in the kidneys down to the bladder to be eliminated.

The reflex areas to the ureter tubes are found in the palms of both hands extending from the kidney reflex in zone 2 at waist level to the bladder reflex in zone 1 just above the wrist.

Kidneys

The two kidneys are situated to the back of the body on either side of the spine at waist level and slightly above and below this level. They are important excretory organs in that they form urine which contains waste products not required by the body and are also important for maintaining the fluid and mineral balance in the body.

The reflex areas to the kidneys are found in the palms of both hands in zones 2 and 3 at waist level and a little above and below waist level.

Adrenal glands

The two adrenals glands are situated just above the kidneys near to the back of the body and just above waist level. They are important hormonal glands and the hormones produced can help reduce inflammation, reduce allergic reactions and also help the body to cope with stress. The hormones can also help with the sodium and water balance in the body, help with the 'fear, flight and fight' responses by the body and there are also additional sex hormones produced by the adrenals.

The reflex areas to the adrenal glands are found in the palms of both hands in zone 2, but on the inner side nearest to zone 1, just above waist level on top of the reflex area to the kidney.

Sciatic nerves

The sciatic nerves are the largest nerves in the body and they start near the lower spine where the lumbar and sacral nerves join together to form a sciatic nerve on each side. The nerves extend down across the buttock and down the back of the leg before dividing in two branches, just above the knee, which then extend down the back of the lower leg.

The reflex areas to the sciatic nerve are found in both hands across just above the wrist, and there is an additional reflex up the sides of both arms.

Backs of the hands

The reflex areas found on the backs of the hands relate mainly to the lymphatic system but also include the reflex areas to the face on the back of the fingers, the reflex areas to the upper and lower limbs along the border on the little-finger side and the reflex areas to the reproductive system in the wrist area.

REFLEX AREAS ABOVE THE LEVEL OF THE SHOULDER GIRDLE AND OVER THE FINGERS

The reflex areas above the level of the shoulder girdle and over the fingers are as follows:

- face

- teeth and gums

- upper lymph nodes and lymph drainage points.

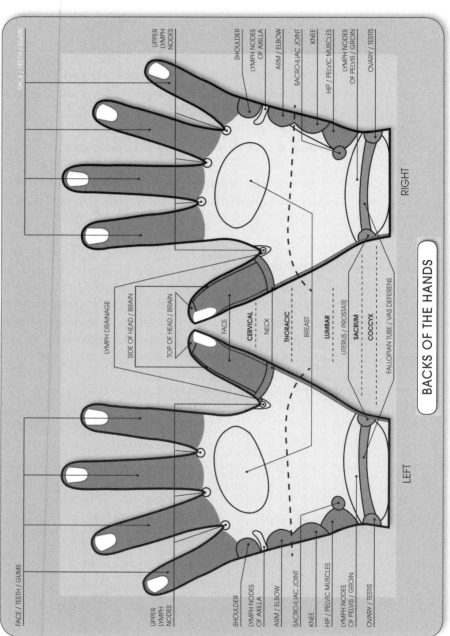

Reflex areas of the backs of the hands

Face

The face is the area to the front of the head and contains the eyes, nose, mouth and throat. It is made up of many muscles and covered by skin.

The reflex areas to the face are found in both hands on the back of the thumb, and on the back of the thumb at the base is the reflex area to the front of the neck and the throat. The face is also represented on the backs of the second, third, fourth and fifth fingers. The reflex areas for the throat including tonsils, adenoids, pharynx and larynx are found at the base of the face area. (These reflex areas are not labelled in the diagram on the previous page.)

Teeth and gums

In the adult there are 32 teeth in the mouth arranged in an upper and lower row with equal pairs of teeth on both sides of the upper and lower rows: the incisors, canines, pre-molars, molars and wisdom teeth. The teeth are important for biting and chewing food at the start of the digestive process. The gums are part of the soft tissue lining of the mouth and they surround the teeth and support them.

The reflex areas to the teeth and the gums are found in both hands on the backs of the second, third, fourth and fifth fingers.

Upper lymph nodes and lymph drainage points

The upper lymph nodes relate to those found in the head and neck areas, and the lymph drainage points relate to where the lymph returns to the bloodstream in the body via the right and left subclavian veins.

The reflex areas to the upper lymph nodes are found in both hands at the base of the webs between the fingers on the backs of the hands. The reflex areas to the lymph drainage points are found in both hands just below the web between the thumb and the second finger on the backs of the hands.

REFLEX AREAS BETWEEN THE LEVELS OF THE
SHOULDER GIRDLE AND THE WAIST

The reflex areas between the levels of the shoulder girdle and the waist are as follows:

- thoracic and abdominal lymphatics

- breasts

- shoulders
- arms
- elbows
- sternum and ribs.

Thoracic and abdominal lymphatics

The lymphatic system is situated throughout the body and is like a secondary circulatory system to the blood. Lymph vessels contain a fluid called lymph and this fluid is eventually returned to the bloodstream via veins in the neck. The lymph vessels drain the excess tissue fluid, but before it is returned to the blood it passes through areas called lymph nodes where cells act to purify the lymph by removing any foreign or damaging substances that might be present. Lymph nodes are situated at various sites in the body including in the head, neck, armpit (axilla), elbow, chest, abdomen, pelvis, groin and knee.

The reflex areas to the lymphatic system are found in both hands occupying most of the area on the backs of the hands.

The thoracic lymphatics refers to the lymph vessels and nodes found in the thorax (chest region). The upper abdominal lymphatics refers to the lymph vessels and nodes found in the upper abdomen in the area between the diaphragm and the waist.

The reflex areas to the thoracic lymphatics are found on the backs of the hands over the metacarpal bones.

The reflex areas to the upper abdominal lymphatics are found on the backs of the hands over the metacarpal bones between the level of the diaphragm and the waist.

Breasts

The breasts (mammary glands) are situated anteriorly in the upper thorax and are present in both women and men. After puberty, breast tissue develops in females due to the female hormones, oestrogen and progesterone, with the main function of preparing the breasts for lactation.

The reflex areas to the breasts are found on the backs of the hands over the upper part of the metacarpal bones mainly in zones 2–4.

Shoulders

The shoulder joint is where the arm attaches to the shoulder girdle of the upper body. This is a ball-and-socket joint with the head of the humerus (the bone of the upper arm) sitting in a socket on the outer side of the shoulder girdle.

The reflex areas to the shoulder joints are found in both hands on the backs of the hands just below the base of the little finger and also (as described previously) in a similar area on the palm side of the hands.

Arms

The two arms are the upper limbs, with the upper arm (the humerus bone) connected to the body via the shoulder joint and the lower arm, or forearm (the radius and ulna bones), attached to the hand at the wrist joint.

The reflex areas for the arms are found in both hands on the backs of the hands from the base of the little finger extending down to waist level in zone 5. The upper arm area is found nearer to the side of the edge of the hand and the forearm and wrist area slightly above this area. The arm is represented as if the elbow is bent with the forearm extending upwards slightly across the front of the chest.

Elbows

The elbow joint is where the upper arm bone (the humerus) joins the lower arm bones (the radius and ulna) and it acts as a hinge joint.

The reflex areas for the elbows are found in both hands on the backs of the hands at waist level.

Sternum and ribs

The sternum (breastbone) is situated centrally in the front of the thorax extending down from the level of the shoulder girdle. There are 12 pairs of ribs and the upper ten pairs attach directly or indirectly to the sternum at the front, and all pairs connect to the thoracic vertebrae at the back.

The reflex area for the sternum is found in both hands in zone 1 on the backs of the hands, close to the lateral border between the level of the shoulder girdle and the diaphragm. The reflex areas for the ribs extend from the sternum area across the five zones between the level of the shoulder girdle and the diaphragm. (These reflex areas are not labelled in the diagram on page 44.)

REFLEX AREAS BELOW WAIST LEVEL

The reflex areas below waist level are as follows:

- lower abdominal lymphatics
- pelvic lymphatics
- knees
- hips
- pelvic muscles
- sacro-iliac joints
- ovaries (in females) and testes (in males)
- fallopian tubes (in females) and vas deferens (in males)
- uterus (in females) and prostate gland (in males).

Lower abdominal and pelvic lymphatics

The lower abdominal lymphatics refers to the lymph vessels and nodes found in the lower abdomen in the area below the waist, and the pelvic lymphatics refers to the lymph vessels and nodes found in the pelvic region.

The reflex areas to the abdominal lymphatics are found on the backs of the hands below waist level, and the reflex areas to the lymph nodes of the pelvis and groin are found on the backs of the hands over the wrist.

Knees

The two knee joints are where the upper and lower leg join, and they are protected at the front by the knee cap. The knee joint is a hinge joint, and many ligaments and cartilages are associated with the joint.

The reflex areas for the knees are found in both hands on the backs of the hands in an area extending from waist level to about halfway down towards the wrist on the medial margin and extending across zone 5. This reflex area also includes the area for the lower leg, ankle and foot.

Hips

The two hip joints are where the upper leg attaches to the body through the pelvis. These are ball-and-socket joints with the head of the femur (the bone of the upper leg) fitting into a socket on the outer side of the pelvic girdle.

The reflex areas for the hips are found in both hands, on the backs of the hands, in an area extending from about halfway down between waist level and the wrist to just above the wrist on the medial margin and extending across zone 5. This reflex area also includes the area for the upper leg (thigh).

Pelvic muscles

The muscles of the pelvis refer to the strong muscles positioned across the buttocks from the sacro-iliac joint to the hip area and the top of the leg.

The reflex areas for the muscles of the pelvis are found in both hands, on the backs of the hands, in an area extending from the hip reflex area (described above) to the sacro-iliac joint reflex area (described below).

Sacro-iliac joints

The two sacro-iliac joints are the areas where the sacrum of the spine joins the ilium of the pelvis, so they are positioned in the lower back area.

The reflex areas for the sacro-iliac joints are found in both hands on the backs of the hands in an area a little way above the wrist in zone 4 (but towards zone 3).

Ovaries and testes

The two ovaries in females are the female reproductive glands which produce the female hormones oestrogen and progesterone, and the ova, the female sex cells. From the time of puberty to the time of menopause, a cycle of events takes place known as the menstrual cycle whereby the hormones are produced in differing amounts to help the development and release of an ovum each month and to act on the other parts of the female reproductive system and in particular, the uterus, to prepare it to receive a fertilised ovum.

The reflex areas for the ovaries are found in both hands in a small dip on the medial (little finger) side of the back of the wrist.

The testes (testicles) in males are the male reproductive glands and are suspended outside the body in the scrotum. The testes produce the sperm, the male sex cells and the male hormone, testosterone, which at puberty develops the male sexual characteristics and maintains these throughout life, though testosterone levels do decrease as men get older.

The reflex areas for the testes are found in both hands in a small dip on the medial (little finger) side of the back of the wrist.

Fallopian tubes and vas deferens

The fallopian tubes (uterine tubes) in females are the tubes that extend from the ovaries on each side of the pelvis to the uterus in the centre of the pelvis. The ova, released at ovulation from the ovaries, travel down the fallopian tubes to the uterus. Fertilisation of an ovum usually takes place in the fallopian tube.

The reflex areas to the fallopian tubes are found in both hands across the backs of the hands above the wrist between the reflex areas for the ovaries and uterus on the sides of the wrist.

The vas deferens in males is one of the tubules along which the sperm travel from the testes to the penis.

The reflex areas to the vas deferens are found in both hands across the backs of the hands above the wrist between the reflex areas for the testes and prostate on the sides of the wrist.

Uterus and prostate gland

The uterus (womb) in females is situated centrally in the pelvic region behind the bladder. It is a muscular pear-shaped organ. From the time of puberty to menopause it goes through a cycle of changes in response to the female hormones to prepare it to receive a fertilised ovum and thus for pregnancy. If fertilisation does not occur, the lining of the uterus is shed together with blood (menstruation) at the end of each menstrual cycle.

The reflex areas for the uterus are found in both hands in a small dip on the lateral (thumb) side of the back of the wrist.

The prostate gland in males is situated just below the bladder and produces a lubricating fluid which helps the transport of sperm.

The reflex areas for the prostate are found in both hands in a small dip on the lateral (thumb side) side of the back of the wrist.

Lateral borders (thumb side) of the hands
SPINE (CERVICAL, THORACIC, LUMBAR, SACRUM, COCCYX)

The spine is made up of bony segments called vertebrae and these can be divided into five regions. The uppermost region is made up of the 7 cervical vertebrae followed by the 12 thoracic vertebrae, the 5 lumbar vertebrae, the 5 sacral vertebrae (fused to form the sacrum) and the 4 coccygeal vertebrae (fused to form the coccyx). The spine surrounds the spinal cord, which is the nerve link between the brain and the rest of the body, so the reflex area relates to both the skeletal and nerve areas.

The reflex areas to the spine are found in both hands all along the lateral border (thumb side) of the hand with the cervical region along the edge of the thumb, then the thoracic region down to waist level, and below waist level the lumbar region followed by the sacrum and then the coccyx, which is found just above the wrist.

The descriptions above cover all the reflex areas in the hands and give descriptions for all the parts of the hands. Most of the main parts of the body are referred to and described above. Those parts that are not referred to by name will still have been treated, since by treating all of both hands, all of the body is treated. In the body there is overlap of certain parts, and the same therefore applies to reflex areas, so in some areas more than one body part is represented. By knowing where all the parts of the body are situated and in which longitudinal and transverse zones they are found, it is possible to determine where in the hand a reflex area to a particular part of the body is found, even if it is not referred to in the descriptions given.

Chapter 5

How to Give Reflexology Treatment to the Hands

To achieve the best results from treatment it is important to work all the reflex areas in both hands. This means that the whole body is treated, which will help maintain or restore balance of all the body systems. Treatment to the reflex areas mainly involves use of the thumb to apply pressure, though the fingers are used to work on certain areas. The precise massage technique to be used is important.

Techniques

There are a number of different techniques used by reflexology practitioners, but the two main approaches considered to be the most effective are the Bayly method and the Ingham method. The Bayly method involves using the thumb to apply pressure and for the thumb to be held bent at the interphalangeal joint and to be kept bent when applying and then releasing the pressure to the reflex point. The lateral side of the thumb near to the tip of the thumb is used to apply pressure, though the medial side can also be used – whichever is most comfortable for the practitioner. (The lateral side of the thumb is the outer side when the body is viewed with the palms of the hands facing forwards.) The pressure is held on each reflex point for just a few seconds and then released, and then the thumb is moved to the next reflex point in the area without lifting the thumb completely off the skin surface. Holding for a few seconds on each point will produce a more fluid movement rather than a 'jabbing' action. The thumb is moved in a forward direction (the direction in which the thumb is pointing) either upwards or across depending on the area being worked.

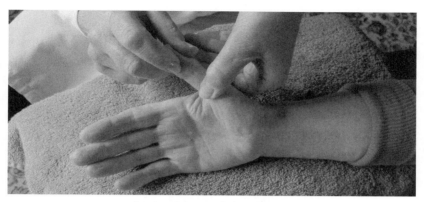

Angle of thumb for treatment

The Ingham method again involves using a bent thumb to apply pressure, but the thumb is then straightened to allow a 'caterpillar-type' movement within the reflex area. This method involves a somewhat faster movement over the reflex points within a reflex area. Another technique sometimes taught involves a circling action on each reflex point.

Different techniques are taught by different training schools, and there is not just one correct way. The important thing is that treatment be given precisely to all the reflex areas and using a technique that is comfortable to the recipient.

Whilst one hand is used to give the massage, the other hand is used to support the area being worked on, and at all times both hands of the practitioner should be in contact with the hand being worked on.

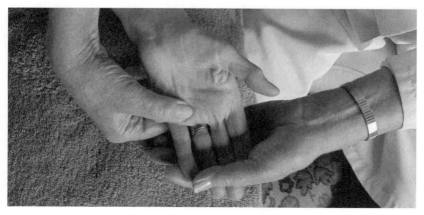

Support of hand for treatment

Position for giving treatment

When giving reflexology treatment to the hands, both practitioner and client will need to be comfortably positioned. The client may be sitting upright in an easy chair, be positioned in a recliner chair as might be used for foot reflexology treatment or might be sitting or lying on a massage couch or bed. The client's hand should be in a relaxed position, and this is best achieved by ensuring that the elbow is slightly bent and the forearm and hand supported on a pillow or cushion with the palm of the hand facing upwards. The practitioner is best positioned alongside the client, so when working the right hand he or she would be seated to the right of the client, and when working the left hand he or she would be seated to the left of the client. The practitioner needs to sit on a chair that enables them to easily reach the hand of the client, which will therefore need to be positioned at about the level of the practitioner's waist. The practitioner will be alongside, but slightly at an angle to, the client. Some practitioners prefer to work sitting facing the client, but this is not so suitable.

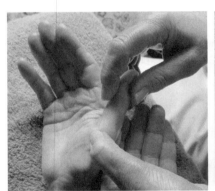
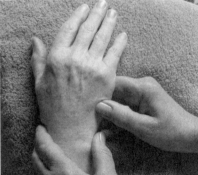
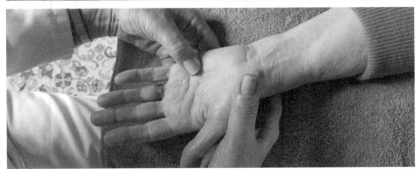

Positions for giving treatment

Treatment procedure

Before the start of treatment, the practitioner should ensure that their hands and fingernails are clean and that all of the fingernails are cut short so that the client does not feel the fingernails when pressure is applied to the reflex areas. A minimum of jewellery on the fingers and wrists should be worn by the practitioner so that this does not interfere with giving treatment. The hands of the client should also be clean, and they should be asked to wash them before treatment if necessary. It is preferable, too, that the client have a minimum of jewellery on the hands and wrists.

Before treatment is commenced, a detailed case history should be taken to enable the practitioner to be aware of any medical conditions present and thereby to know which reflex areas will be the most important for this client and which areas will require extra attention. It will also ensure that should a medical condition be present that is not appropriate to treat, then treatment would not be carried out.

It should be explained to the client what they may feel as the treatment is given. They will be aware of pressure as the massage is applied, but in some areas it might feel as if more pressure is being applied and that there is a degree of sensitivity. Pressure should always be adjusted by the practitioner, though, so that treatment is not uncomfortable, but there may be some areas of tenderness. In some areas 'grittiness' might be felt and this might indicate a degree of imbalance in the corresponding body area. These 'gritty' areas are sometimes described as being deposits of a crystalline substance, but this has not been proven. In general, if a client has experienced foot reflexology, they may not experience as much sensitivity in the reflex areas of the hand as in those found in the feet, though in some cases the opposite occurs with a client being more aware of the sensitivity of the reflex areas in the hands than those in the feet. The fact that generally there is less sensitivity may be because the hands are used for many more different tasks than the feet and therefore are more used to pressure being applied to them by the various activities that they may perform.

Before working on the precise reflex areas, the practitioner should have a look at the client's hands and take note of the general condition of the hands including the skin texture and colour, the muscle tone in the hands, the bone structure and the condition of the nails. The condition of the hands may reflect a problem in the body represented by the underlying reflex area.

When first touching the client's hands the temperature will also be observed, with cold hands suggesting poor circulation and hot, perspiring hands suggesting a possible glandular imbalance. Some general massage to the hand might be given initially to allow the client to get used to the practitioner touching their hand and to warm the hand if it is a bit cold.

If the skin of the client's hands is very dry, a light, non-greasy, unperfumed, hypoallergenic cream might be gently rubbed into the hands. Any cream used should be readily absorbed and not leave the hand too greasy which would not allow treatment to be given precisely to each reflex area. If the skin of the client's hand is a bit moist and sweaty, a light dusting of unperfumed powder (such as calendula powder) might be gently rubbed onto the hands which would then allow the practitioner to work precisely on the reflex areas without slipping. However, in most cases it is not necessary to use either cream or powder when working on the reflex areas in the hands.

Order of treatment

It is advisable to follow a specific order to treat the reflex areas in the hands. By following a specific order, this will become an automatic routine for the practitioner and ensure that all the reflex areas in both hands are worked precisely. The order of treatment which follows is that taught by the Bayly School of Reflexology, though it can always be adapted. This system involves working first on the right hand and then the left hand with a few relaxation exercises applied at the end of working all the reflex areas in each hand. Extra attention to important reflex areas for the individual client is usually given having worked all the reflex areas in the hand, though additional massage might be given to these areas whilst going through the order. (The position of the reflex areas is described in Chapter 4.)

Right hand

PITUITARY

Using the right thumb, apply pressure to the centre of the thumb. Work from over the top of the thumb and use the left hand to support the base of the thumb. Having worked the very centre of the thumb, work a square area all around the centre point, and this will relate to other parts of the centre of the brain.

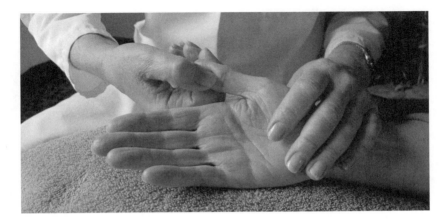

NECK

Using the left thumb, start on the lateral border of the hand and work across zone 1 towards zone 2 just above where the thumb joins the palm of the hand. Support the top of the thumb with the right hand.

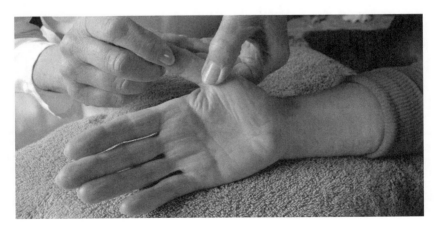

SIDE OF HEAD/BRAIN

Using the left thumb, work up the side of the thumb (the side next to the second finger) from the base of thumb to the tip. It is best to turn the client's thumb so that the back of the thumb is facing you.

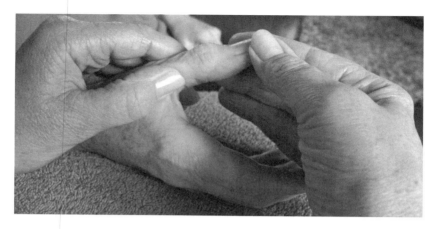

TOP OF HEAD/BRAIN

Change hands at the top of the thumb and using the right thumb work over the top of the thumb starting from the second-finger side. Repeat this movement several times but each time working across a little further down from the top of the thumb.

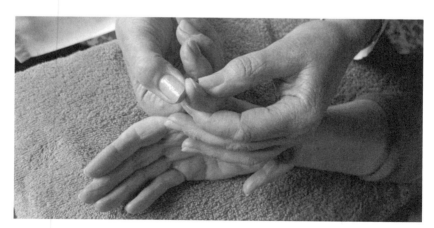

SPINE

Using the right thumb, work down the lateral side of the hand straight down to the just above the wrist, then change hands and come back up the spine reflex using the left thumb up the side of the hand. The right hand should support the thumb as you work back up the spine reflex.

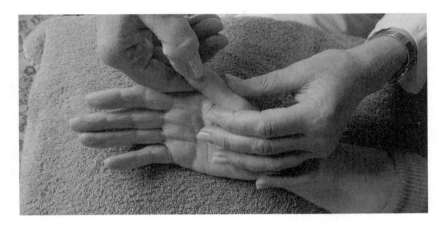

FACE

Using the left thumb, work the area on the back of the thumb working from the base of the thumb to just below the nail. Support the top of the thumb with the right hand and turn the client's thumb so that the back of the thumb is facing you.

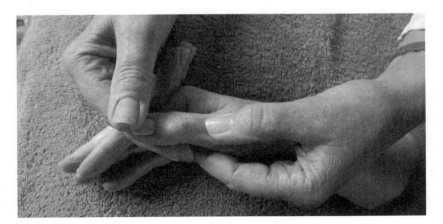

SINUSES

For the sinuses in the fingers, each finger has to be worked on in turn starting with the second finger. Support the finger at the tip using the right hand and with the left thumb work from the base of the finger up to the tip. Then work up the side of the finger on the lateral side. Follow the same sequence for each finger in turn. One movement up the palm side and the finger side should be sufficient, but if you are working on very broad fingers you might need to work with more movements.

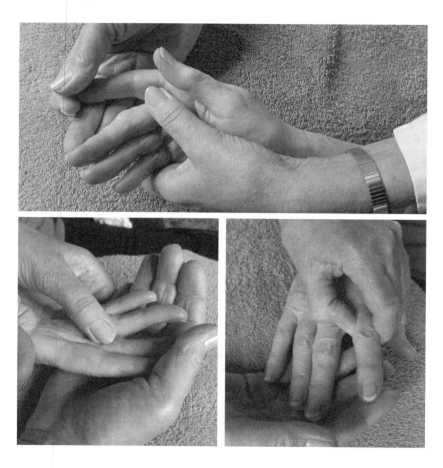

TEETH AND GUMS

For the teeth and gums, each finger has to be worked on in turn starting with the second finger. Turn the hand over so that the back of the hand is facing you. Support the finger at the tip using the right hand and with the left thumb work from the base of the finger up to the tip just below the nail. Then work up the medial border of each finger (sinuses). Follow the same sequence for each finger in turn.

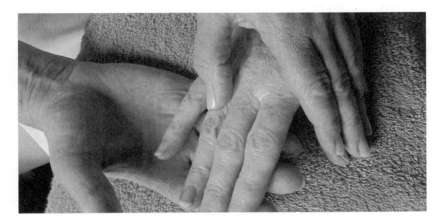

EYE

Using the right thumb, work just below where the second and third fingers join the palm of the hand from zone 2 to zone 3. Use the left hand to straighten and pull back the fingers slightly.

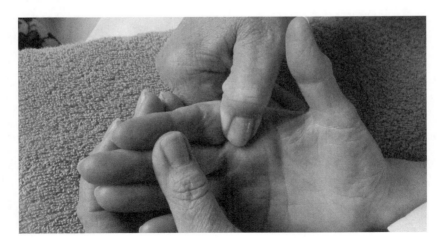

EUSTACHIAN TUBE

Work with the right or left thumb on the point just below the web between the third and fourth fingers in the palm of the hand.

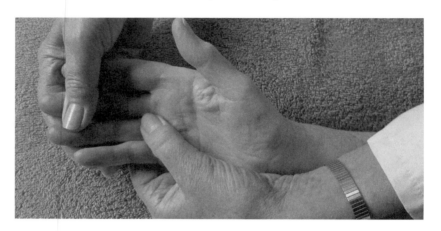

EAR

Using the right thumb, work just below where the fourth and fifth fingers join the palm of the hand from zone 4 to zone 5. Use the left hand to straighten and pull back the fingers slightly. (If working on a large hand, it might be easier to work this area using the left thumb from zones 5 to 4.)

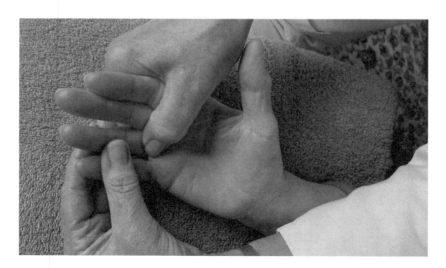

SHOULDER

Using the left thumb, work the area in the palm of the hand beneath the little finger and also on the side and back of the hand around the base of the little finger.

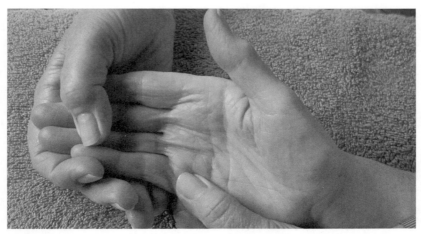

Palm of hand

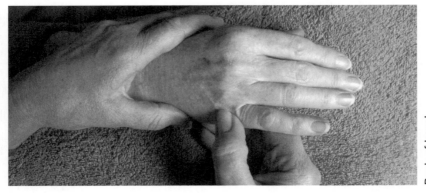

Back of hand

ARM AND ELBOW

Have the back of the hand facing you and with the right thumb work down the medial border of the back of the hand from the shoulder reflex to waist level (about halfway down the back of the hand). This area relates to the arm and the elbow. Come back up the same area using the left thumb but working a little higher on the back of the hand than when you worked down. The area just below the fingers relates to the wrist.

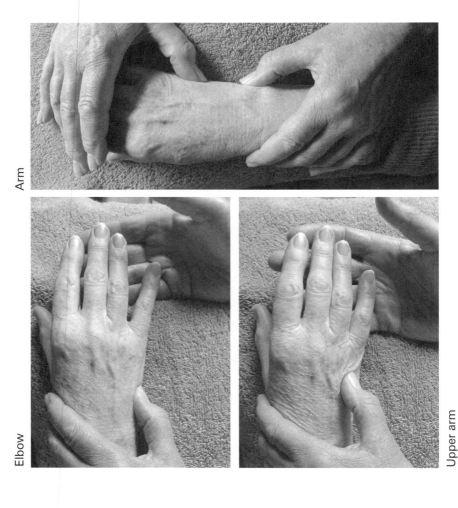

Arm

Elbow

Upper arm

THYROID AND PARATHYROIDS

Using the left thumb, work across the area just below where the thumb joins the palm of the hand from the side of the hand towards the border with zone 2. Repeat this movement three or four times working a little lower down each time. As you work this area you will overlap the parathyroid reflexes on the edge of zone 1 next to zone 2 with the upper parathyroid reflex at the upper part of the area and the lower parathyroid reflex at the base of the area.

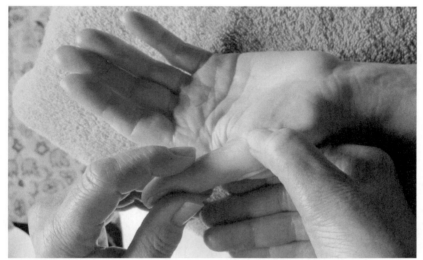

Thyroid

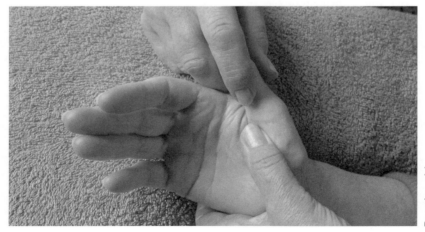

Parathyroid

LUNG

Using the right thumb, start in zone 2 in the palm of the hand below the second finger and work straight across all the zones towards zone 5. When you get to zone 5, change hands and come back with the left thumb across all the zones again but a little lower than worked before. Keep working across the area, changing hands as you get to the side of hand and working a little lower down the palm each time until you have worked all the area relating to the lung.

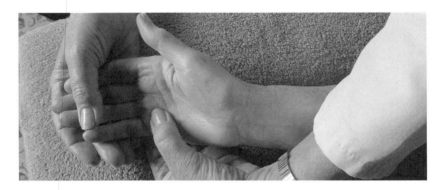

SOLAR PLEXUS

Using the left or right thumb, work the area in zones 2 and 3 just below diaphragm level, which is approximately where a crease mark starts in zone 5 of the palm of the hand about 1–2 cm down from the fifth finger and extends across all the zones from this line.

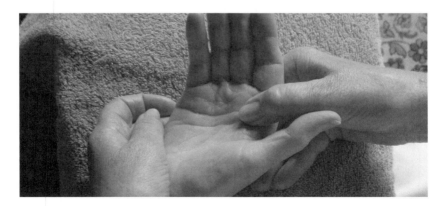

LIVER

Using the left thumb, start in zone 5 just below diaphragm level and work across all of the zones, then change hands when you get to the inner border of the hand and use the right thumb to come back across the zones following a slightly lower line across the hand. Repeat these movements for the rest of the liver area but not working so far over on the inner side of the hand, with each movement with the lower part of the liver reflex being just in zones 5, 4 and 3.

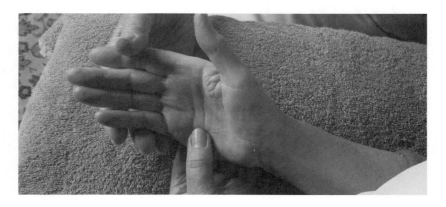

GALL BLADDER

As you work the lower part of the liver area you will overlap the gall bladder reflex area, but this small area will also be worked using the left thumb on the precise point in zone 3 just above waist level.

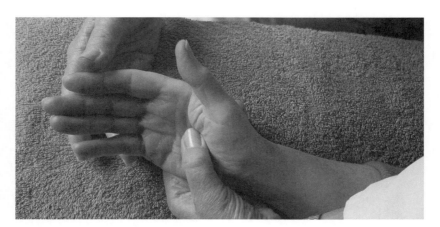

STOMACH AND PANCREAS

The area between the diaphragm and the waist in zone 1 relates to the stomach and the pancreas, with the stomach in the whole area and the pancreas in the lower half of the area. Using the right thumb, work across this area starting on the medial side of the hand, and then repeat the same movement a little lower down the palm.

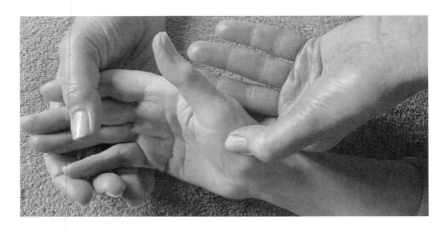

SMALL INTESTINE

Using the right thumb, start in zone 1 just below waist level and work across to zone 4, then change hands and use the left thumb to come back across the zones following a slightly lower line in that region. Continue similarly across the hand to just above the wrist finishing in zones 4 and 5.

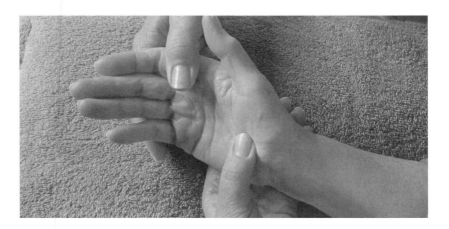

ILEO-CAECAL VALVE

Using the left thumb, work just above the wrist in zones 4 and 5.

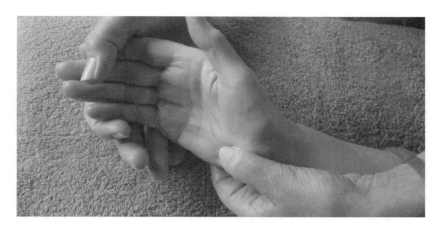

ASCENDING COLON

Using the left thumb, work up from the ileo-caecal valve, up the ascending colon reflex to waist level.

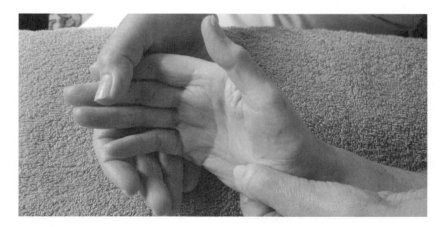

TRANSVERSE COLON

Using the left hand, work across all the zones at waist level from zones 4 and 5 to zone 1.

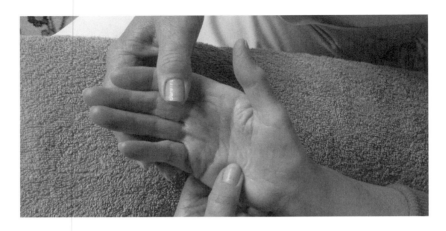

BLADDER

Using the left thumb, work an area on the back of the hand and around the side of the hand into the palm of the hand a short distance above the wrist.

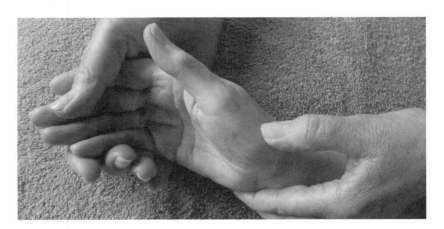

URETER TUBE

Using the left thumb, work upwards and outwards from the bladder reflex in zone 1 to the kidney reflex in zone 2 at waist level.

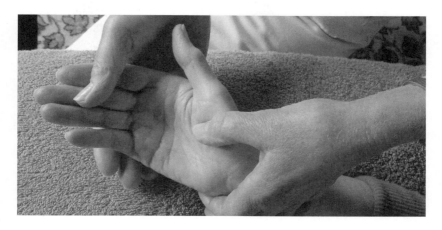

KIDNEY

Using the left thumb, work zones 2 and 3 at waist level, and below and above waist level.

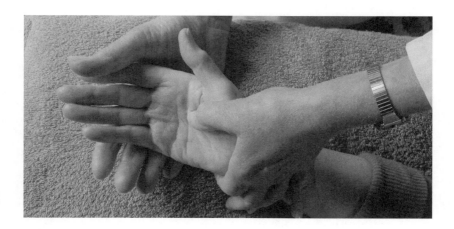

ADRENAL

Using the left thumb, work in zone 2 just above the kidney reflex and slightly more towards zone 1.

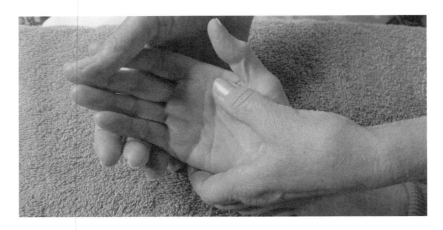

SCIATIC LOOP (PLUS UP-PALM SIDE OF ARM)

Work the area just above the wrist either with the right hand working from zone 1 to zone 5 or with the left hand from zone 5 to zone 1. Then continue the sciatic nerve reflex up the sides of the arm using the fingers or thumb of the right hand on either side of the arm, with the palm of the hand facing upwards, for about 10 cm up the arm. Then use a gentle pinching action to come down this area on the arm.

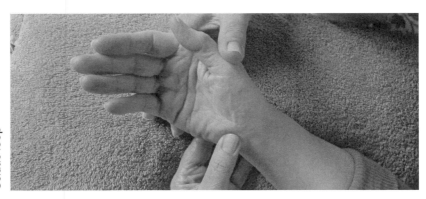

Sciatic loop

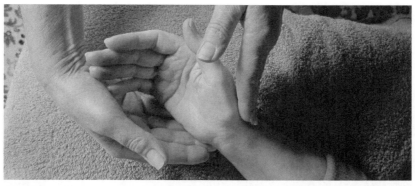

Sciatic (upper)

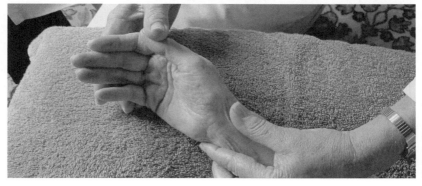

Sciatic (lower)

KNEE

Have the back of the hand upwards. Using the right thumb, work an area from waist level on the little-finger side of the hand to halfway towards the wrist working at right angles to the side of the hand from zone 5 to zone 4, and then repeat this movement a little lower towards the wrist each time.

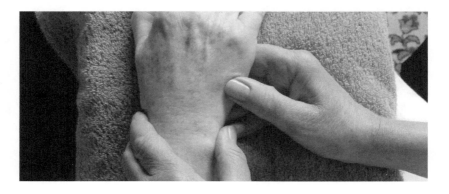

HIP

Using the right thumb, work an area from the knee reflex to just above the wrist working at right angles to the side of the hand from zone 5 to zone 4, and then repeat this movement a little lower towards the wrist each time.

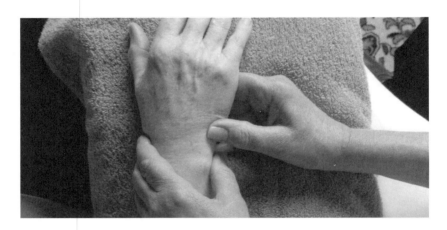

PELVIC MUSCLES

Using the right thumb, work an area on the back of the hand from the hip area across to the sacro-iliac joint area in zone 4.

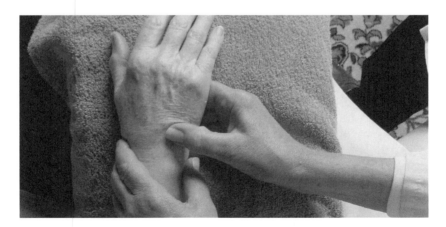

SACRO-ILIAC JOINT

Using the right thumb, work an area on the back of the hand about in line with the fourth finger and a short distance above the wrist.

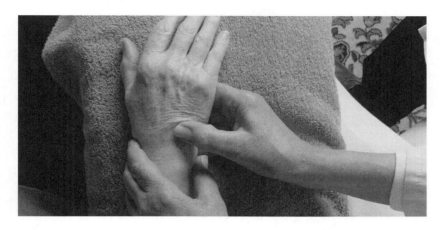

OVARY OR TESTIS

Using the left thumb, work a point just above the wrist on the medial side of the hand in a small dip slightly on the back of the hand.

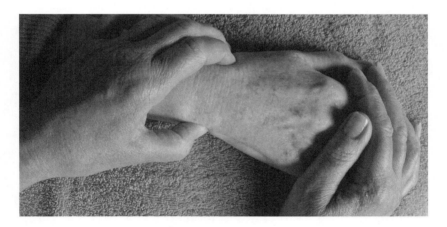

FALLOPIAN TUBE OR VAS DEFERENS

Using the right thumb, work over the back of the hand, just above the wrist, from the ovary/testis reflex on the medial side to the uterus/prostate point on the lateral side.

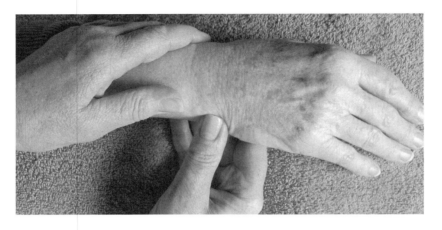

UTERUS OR PROSTATE

Using the left thumb, work a point just above the wrist on the lateral side of the hand in a small dip slightly on the back of the hand.

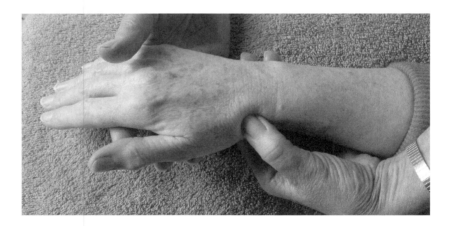

LYMPHATIC SYSTEM (PLUS BREAST)

Using the right thumb, work the back of the hand from the web between the fingers down to just above the wrist. Start on the inner side of the hand at the web between the thumb and second finger. Having done all the areas on the back of the hand, you will have overlapped the breast reflex just above diaphragm level in zones 2–4. Work the reflex areas for the lymphatics of the pelvis and the groin by working over the wrist.

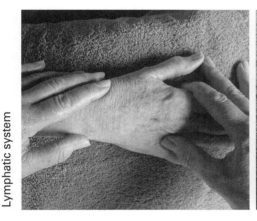

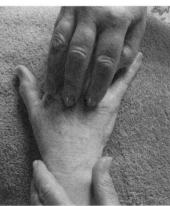

Lymphatic system

Breast

LYMPHATIC DRAINAGE

Using the right thumb and second finger, pinch between the thumb and the second finger and pull away from the hand.

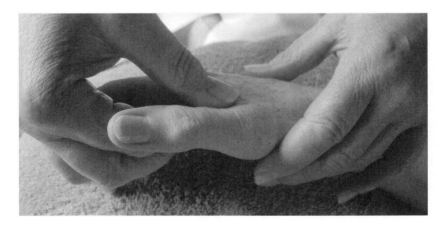

ROTATION OF FINGERS

Use the left hand to support the base of the right thumb joint from the lateral margin of the hand and use the thumb and second finger of the right hand to hold the thumb from over the tip of the thumb, gripping near to the base of the thumb. Then rotate the thumb gently a few times in one direction and a few times in the other direction. Using the hands in the same position, rotate all of the other fingers individually.

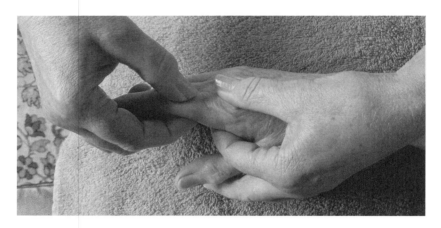

'WRINGING' OF HAND

Place the left hand round the little finger side of the hand with the fingers on the back of the hand and the thumb on the palm side, and place the right hand similarly round the thumb side of the hand. 'Wring' the hands so as to spread apart the bones of the hand.

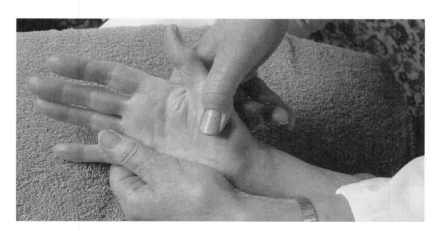

'KNEADING' OF HAND

Using the flat surface of a clenched fist, press up at diaphragm level in the palm of the hand, put the other hand flat on the back of the hand and press the hands against each other rotating both at the same time.

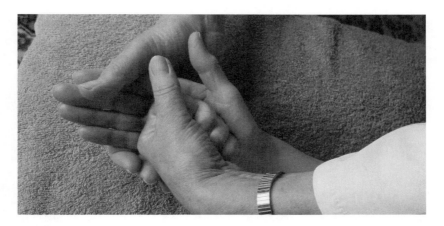

ROTATION OF WRIST

With the palm of the hand facing upwards, place the left hand over the wrist, use the right hand to support the fingers and rotate the wrist a few times in one direction and then the other direction.

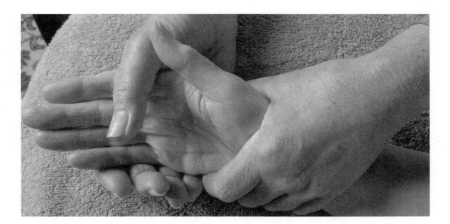

SOLAR PLEXUS BREATHING

Place the left thumb on the solar plexus reflex in the palm of the right hand and support the back of the fingers with the right hand. Apply pressure to the reflex as the patient takes a deep breath in, and at the same time ease the fingers towards the palm side of the hand slightly, then as they breathe out ease the pressure off the solar plexus reflex and ease the fingers back. Repeat three or four times.

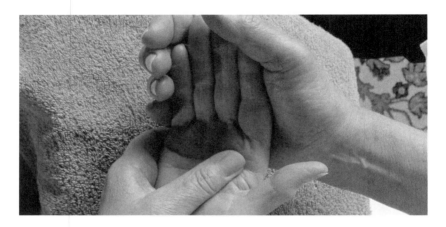

Left hand
PITUITARY

Using the left thumb, apply pressure to the centre of the thumb. Work from over the top of the thumb and use the right hand to support the base of the thumb. Having worked the very centre of the thumb, work a square area all around the centre point and this will relate to other parts of the centre of the brain.

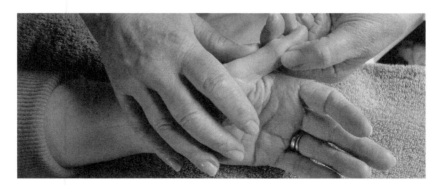

NECK

Using the right thumb, start on the lateral border of the hand and work across zone 1 towards zone 2 just above where the thumb joins the palm of the hand. Support the top of the thumb with the left hand.

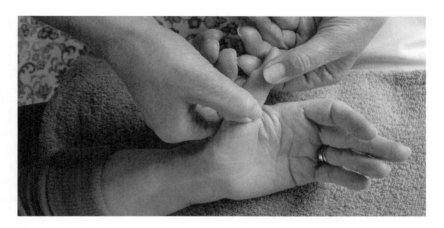

SIDE OF HEAD AND SIDE OF BRAIN

Using the right thumb, work up the side of the thumb (the side next to the second finger) from the base of the thumb to the tip. It is best to turn the client's thumb so that the back of the thumb is facing you.

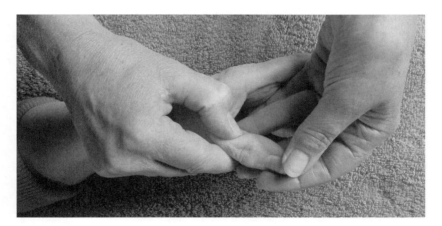

TOP OF HEAD AND TOP OF BRAIN

Change hands at the top of the thumb and using the left thumb work over the top of the thumb starting from the second-finger side. Repeat this movement several times but each time working across a little further down from the top of the thumb.

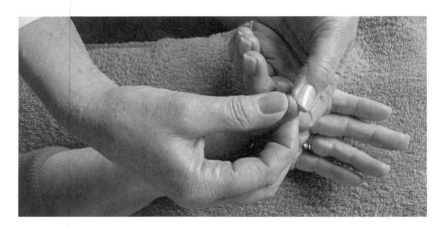

SPINE

Using the left thumb, work down the lateral side of the hand straight down to just above the wrist, then change hands and come back up the spine reflex using the right thumb up the side of the hand. The left hand should support the thumb as you work back up the spine reflex.

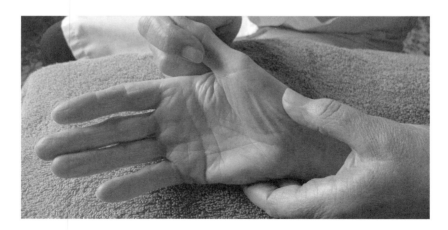

FACE

Using the right thumb, work the area on the back of the thumb working from the base of the thumb to just below the nail. Support the top of the thumb with the left hand and turn the client's thumb so that the back of the thumb is facing you.

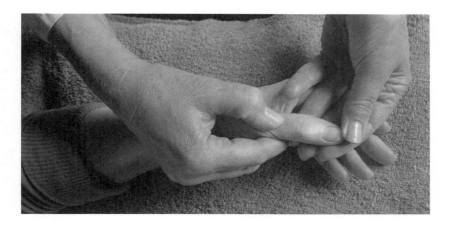

SINUSES

For the sinuses in the fingers, each finger has to be worked on in turn starting with the second finger. Support the finger at the tip using the left hand and with the right thumb work from the base of the finger up to the tip. Then work up the side of the finger on the lateral side. Follow the same sequence for each finger in turn. One movement up the palm side and the finger side should be sufficient, but if you are working on very broad fingers you might need to work with more movements.

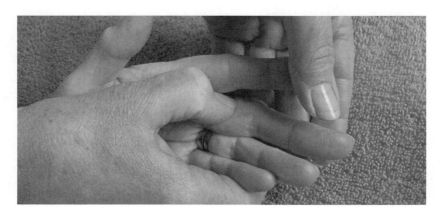

TEETH AND GUMS

For the teeth and gums, each finger has to be worked on in turn starting with the second finger. Turn the hand over so that the back of the hand is facing you. Support the finger at the tip using the left hand and with the right thumb work from the base of the finger up to the tip just below the nail. Then work up the medial border of each finger (sinuses). Follow the same sequence for each finger in turn.

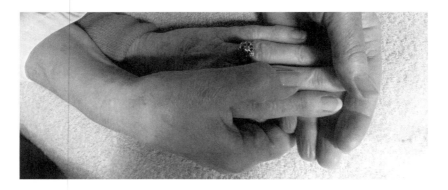

EYE

Using the left thumb, work just below where the second and third fingers join the palm of the hand from zone 2 to zone 3. Use the right hand to straighten and pull back the fingers slightly.

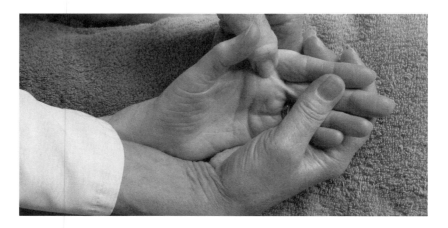

EUSTACHIAN TUBE

Work with the left thumb on the point just below the web between the third and fourth fingers in the palm of the hand.

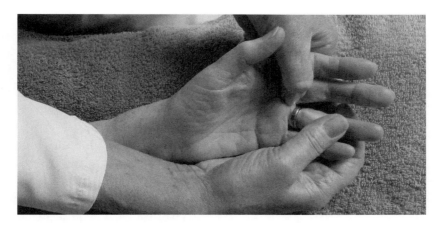

EAR

Using the left thumb, work just below where the fourth and fifth fingers join the palm of the hand from zone 4 to zone 5. Use the right hand to straighten and pull back the fingers slightly. (If working on a large hand, it might be easier to work this area using the right thumb from zones 5 to 4.)

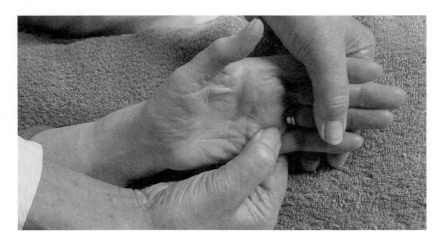

SHOULDER

Using the right thumb, work the area in the palm of the hand beneath the little finger and also on the side and back of the hand around the base of the little finger.

Palm of hand

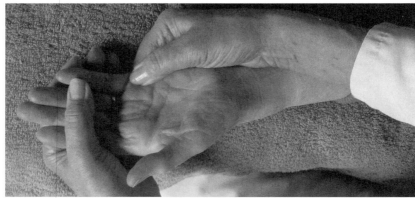

Back of hand

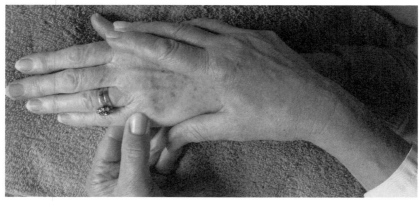

ARM AND ELBOW

Have the back of the hand facing you and with the left thumb work down the medial border of the back of the hand from the shoulder reflex to waist level (about halfway down the back of the hand). This area relates to the arm and the elbow. Come back up the same area using the right thumb but working a little higher on the back of the hand than when you worked down. The area just below the fingers relates to the wrist.

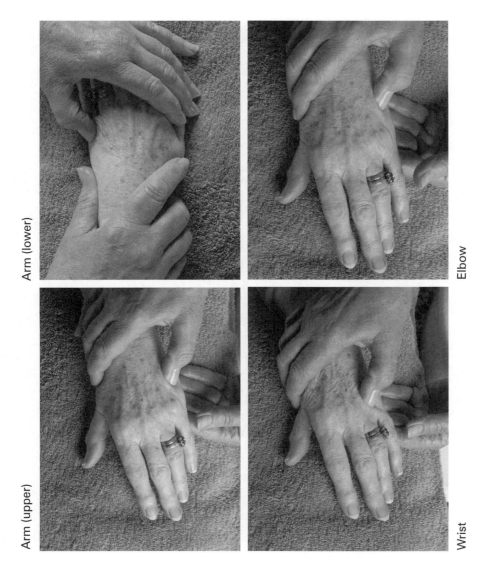

Arm (lower)

Elbow

Arm (upper)

Wrist

THYROID AND PARATHYROIDS

Using the right thumb, work across the area just below where the thumb joins the palm of the hand from the side of the hand towards the border with zone 2. Repeat this movement three or four times working a little lower down each time. As you work this area you will overlap the parathyroid reflexes on the edge of zone 1 next to zone 2 with the upper parathyroid reflex at the upper part of the area and the lower parathyroid reflex at the base of the area.

Thyroid

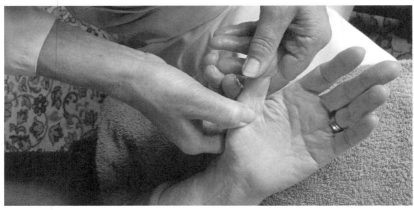

Parathyroids

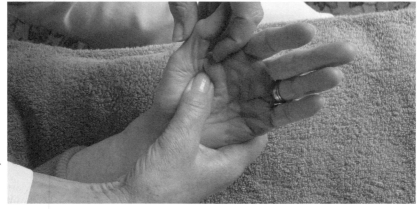

LUNG

Using the left thumb, start in zone 2 in the palm of the hand below the second finger and work straight across all the zones toward zone 5. When you get to zone 5, change hands and come back with the right thumb across all the zones again but a little lower than worked before. Keep working across the area, changing hands as you get to the side of the hand and working a little lower down the palm each time until you have worked all the area relating to the lung, but in the lower part of this area work zones 4 and 5, leaving a space for the heart reflex in zones 2 and 3.

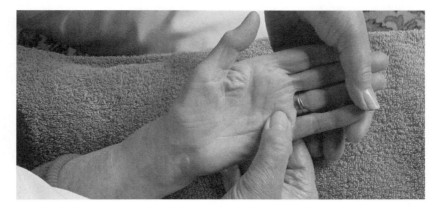

HEART

Using the right thumb, work the area in zones 2 and 3 just above diaphragm level.

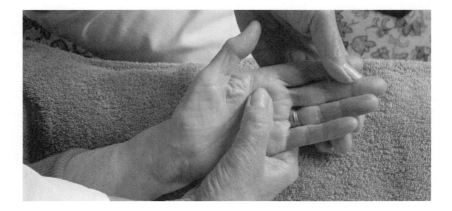

SOLAR PLEXUS

Using the right thumb, work the area in zones 2 and 3 just below diaphragm level, which is approximately where a crease mark starts in zone 5 of the palm of the hand about 1–2 cm down from the fifth finger and extends across all the zones from this line.

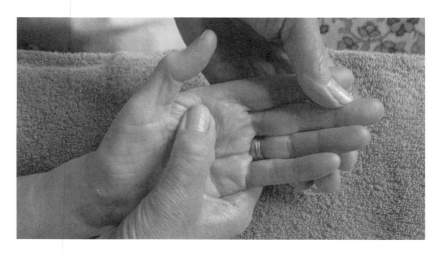

SPLEEN

Using the right thumb, work from zone 5 to zone 4 filling in the area between the diaphragm and the waist.

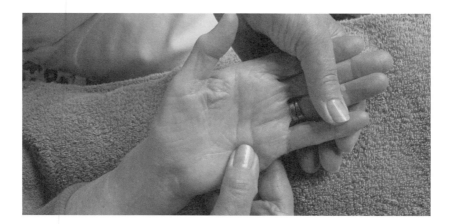

STOMACH AND PANCREAS

The area between the diaphragm and the waist in zones 1–3 relates to the stomach and the pancreas, with the stomach in the whole area and the pancreas in the lower half of the area. Using the left thumb, work across these areas from zone 1 to zone 3 or with the right thumb from zone 3 to zone 1 repeating the same movement each time a little lower down the palm.

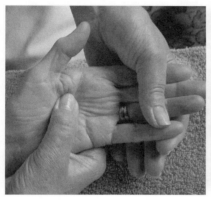
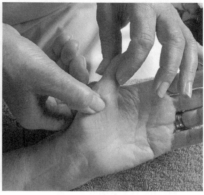

Stomach

Pancreas

SMALL INTESTINE

Using the left thumb, start in zone 1 just below waist level and work across to zone 4, then change hands and use the right thumb to come back across the zones following a slightly lower line in that region. Continue similarly across the hand to just above the wrist, finishing in zones 4 and 5.

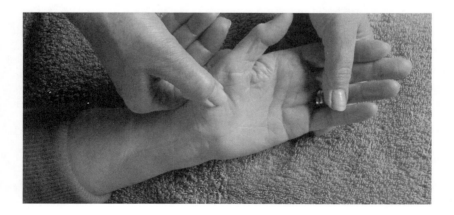

TRANSVERSE COLON

Using the left thumb, work across all the zones at waist level from zone 1 to zones 4 and 5.

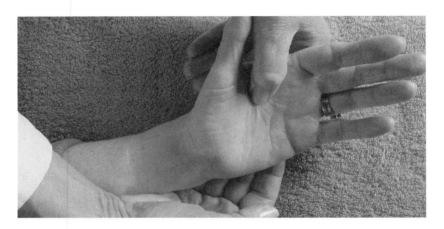

DESCENDING COLON

Using the left thumb, work down from waist level in zones 4 and 5 to just above the wrist.

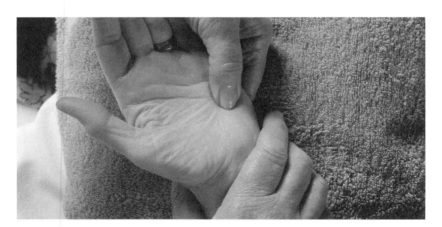

SIGMOID COLON AND RECTUM

Using the right thumb, work from zones 4 and 5 just above the wrist across the palm of the hand to zone 1 (rectum).

Sigmoid colon

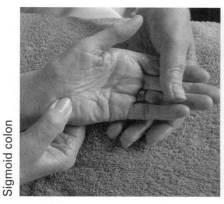 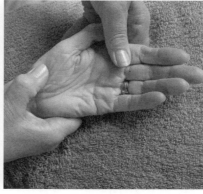

Rectum

BLADDER

Using the left thumb, work an area on the back of the hand and around the side of the hand into the palm of the hand a short distance above the wrist.

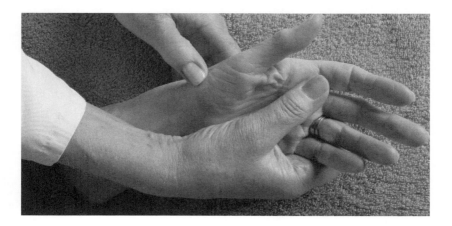

URETER TUBE

Using the left thumb, work upwards and outwards from the bladder reflex in zone 1 to the kidney reflex in zone 2 at waist level.

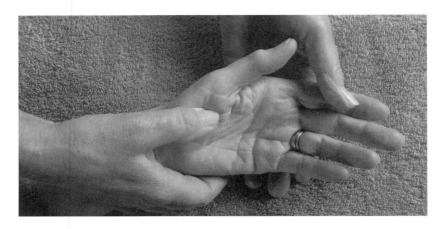

KIDNEY

Using the left thumb, work zones 2 and 3 at waist level, and below and above waist level.

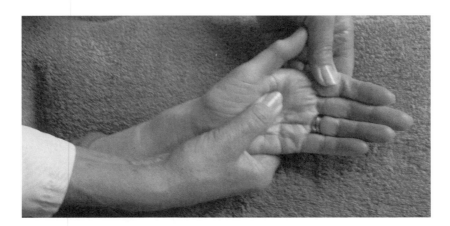

ADRENAL

Using the left or right thumb, work in zone 2 just above the kidney reflex and slightly more towards zone 1.

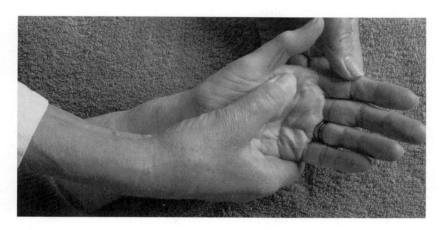

SCIATIC LOOP (PLUS UP-PALM SIDE OF ARM)

Work the area just above the wrist either with the right hand working from zone 1 to zone 5 or with the left hand from zone 5 to zone 1. Continue the sciatic nerve reflex up the sides of the arm using the fingers or thumb of the left hand on either side of the arm, with the palm of the hand facing upwards, for about 10 cm up the arm. Then use a gentle pinching action to come down this area on the arm.

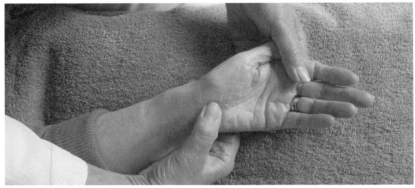

Sciatic loop

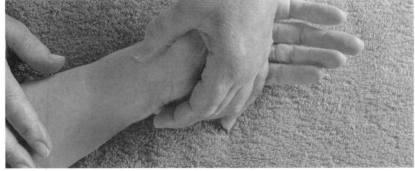

Sciatic (upper)

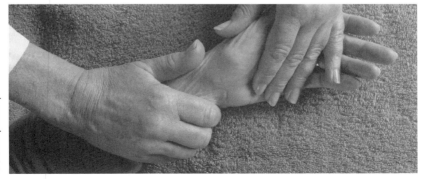

Sciatic (lower)

KNEE

Have the back of the hand upwards. Using the left or right thumb, work an area from waist level on the little-finger side of the hand to halfway towards the wrist, working at right angles to the side of the hand from zone 5 to zone 4, and then repeat this movement a little lower towards the wrist each time.

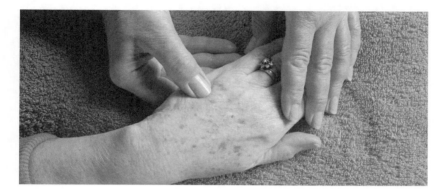

HIP

Using the left or right thumb, work an area from the knee reflex to just above the wrist, working at right angles to the side of hand from zone 5 to zone 4, and then repeat this movement a little lower towards the wrist each time.

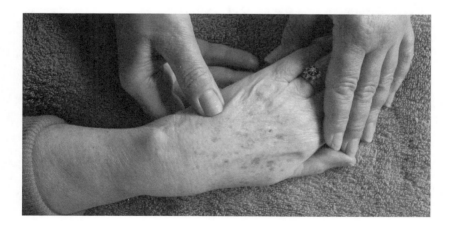

PELVIC MUSCLES

Using the left or right thumb, work an area on the back of the hand from the hip area across to the sacro-iliac joint area in zone 4.

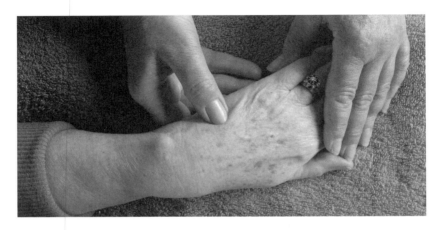

SACRO-ILIAC JOINT

Using the left or right thumb, work an area on the back of the hand about in line with the fourth finger and a short distance above the wrist.

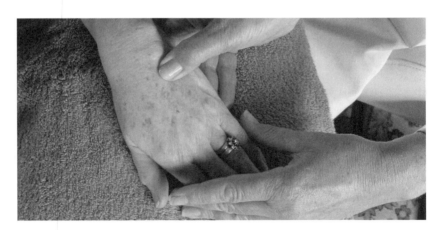

OVARY OR TESTIS

Using the left thumb, work a point just above the wrist on the medial side of the hand in a small dip slightly on the back of the hand.

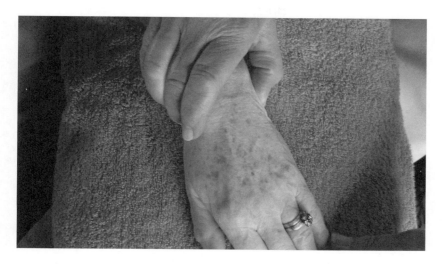

FALLOPIAN TUBE OR VAS DEFERENS

Using the left thumb, work over the back of the hand, just above the wrist, from the ovary/testis reflex on the medial side to the uterus/prostate point on the lateral side.

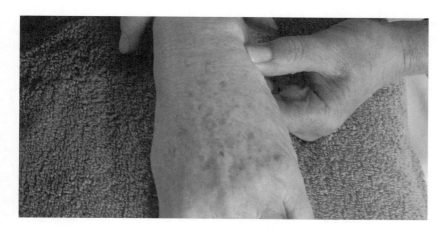

UTERUS OR PROSTATE

Using the right thumb, work a point just above the wrist on the lateral side of the hand in a small dip slightly on the back of the hand.

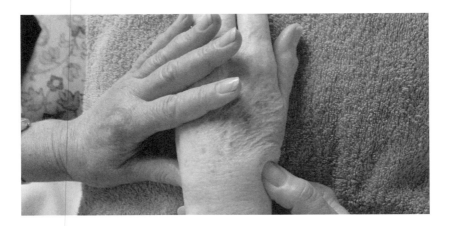

LYMPHATIC SYSTEM (PLUS BREAST)

Using the left thumb, work the back of the hand from the web between the fingers down to just above the wrist. Start on the inner side of the hand at the web between the thumb and second finger. Having done all the areas on the back of the hand, you will have overlapped the breast reflex just above diaphragm level in zones 2–4. Work the reflex areas for the lymphatics of the pelvis and the groin by working over the wrist.

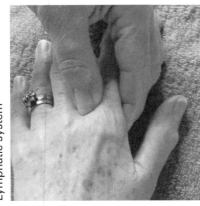

Lymphatic system

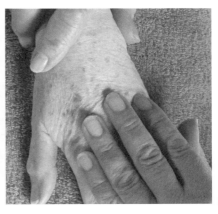

Breast

LYMPHATIC DRAINAGE

Using the left thumb and second finger, pinch between the thumb and the second finger, and pull away from the hand.

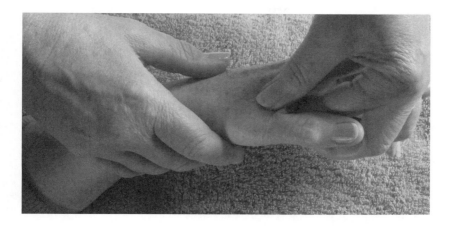

ROTATION OF FINGERS

Use the right hand to support the base of the left thumb joint from the lateral margin of the hand, and use the thumb and second finger of the left hand to hold the thumb from over the tip of the thumb gripping near to the base of the thumb. Then rotate the thumb gently a few times in one direction and a few times in the other direction. Using the hands in the same position, rotate all of the other fingers individually.

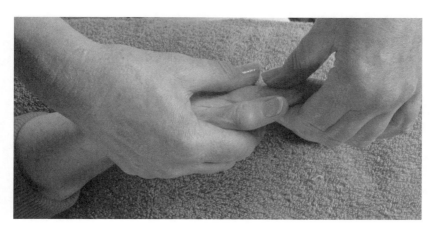

'WRINGING' OF HAND

Place the right hand round the little-finger side of the hand with the fingers on the back of the hand and the thumb on the palm side, and place the left hand similarly round the thumb side of the hand. 'Wring' the hands so as to spread apart the bones of the hand.

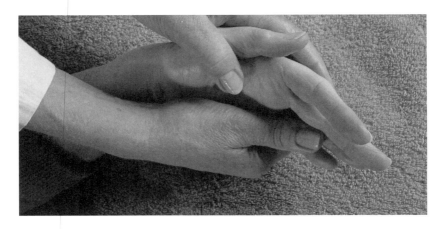

'KNEADING' OF HAND

Using the flat surface of a clenched fist, press up at diaphragm level in the palm of the hand, put the other hand flat on the back of the hand and press the hands against each other rotating both at the same time.

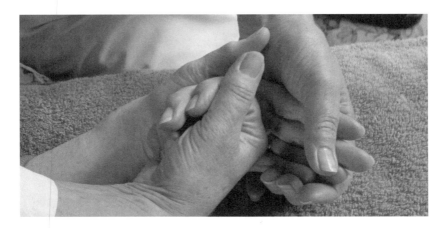

ROTATION OF WRIST

With the palm of the hand facing upwards, place the right hand over the wrist, use the left hand to support the fingers and rotate the wrist a few times in one direction and then the other direction.

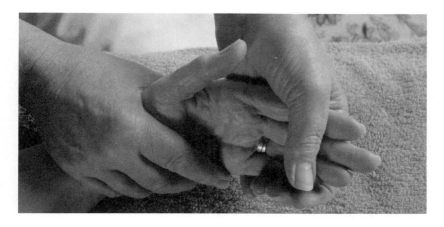

SOLAR PLEXUS BREATHING

Place the right thumb on the solar plexus reflex in the palm of the left hand and support the back of the fingers with the left hand. Apply pressure to the reflex as the patient takes a deep breath in and at the same time ease the fingers towards the palm side of the hand slightly, then as they breathe out ease the pressure off the solar plexus reflex and ease the fingers back. Repeat three or four times.

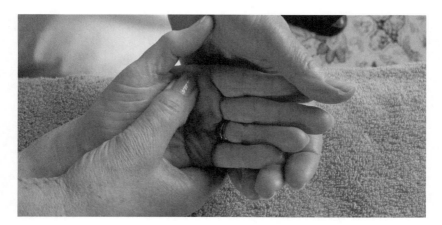

A hand reflexology treatment lasts on average about 40 minutes, though obviously this depends on the size of the hands and whether it is necessary to rework a number of reflex areas. When the treatment is complete, the practitioner should wash his or her hands. The client should be offered a glass of water following treatment – this is particularly important if they are feeling thirsty – and they should also be advised of any possible reactions that might be expected as a result of treatment.

Possible reactions to treatment

As a result of treatment it is possible sometimes for reactions to treatment to occur. Provided that treatment has been given correctly with the correct amount of pressure and for the correct amount of time, thereby not overworking, it is unlikely that these reactions will be too severe. These reactions would normally occur after a first or second treatment in a course of treatment.

Some of the possible reactions to treatment include increased elimination from the eliminatory organs as unwanted toxins are removed from the body. These are positive signs and careful treatment should prevent them from being too severe and debilitating to the client. The reactions would occur within about 24 to 48 hours of treatment and should disappear in a similar time. They would involve increased elimination from the system where congestion is present. The types of reaction that might be experienced could include:

- With the respiratory system, increased secretions of mucous membranes of the nose to give a runny nose and sneezing; increased secretion of the mucous membranes of the pharynx and the bronchi leading to coughing and maybe coughing up mucus; popping in the ears if they are blocked; altered noises experienced by the tinnitus sufferer; a nose bleed after treatment, which if it is not severe, can often cause relief of a blocked nose.

- With the urinary system, increased excretion of urine, and the urine might have a different odour or colour.

- With the digestive system, increased activity of the bowels with an increase in frequency, volume and bulk of the stools, flatulence, nausea (it is best that a client not eat a heavy meal before treatment as this might increase the likelihood of this reaction) and headaches (as the liver is stimulated to increase elimination of toxins).

- With the skin, increased perspiration, worsening of a skin rash and appearance of spots on the skin.

Other possible reactions include:

- With arthritis, there may be more pain experienced in the affected joint for about 24 hours.

- With sleep, there may be disturbed sleep and an increased awareness of dreams, though more commonly there is improved sleep. Often a client can feel quite tired after treatment acting as a reminder that rest is needed. They might also find themselves yawning a lot after treatment.

- With women, there might be an increased vaginal discharge which may be more acidic causing inflammation and irritation.

- With emotions, there might be feelings of depression, increased sensitivity and bad temper, though more usually there is a feeling of calmness and well-being.

Additionally, sometimes conditions that have been present in the past but have been treated by suppressing, rather than by treating the condition, may flare up.

Frequency of treatment

In most cases, reflexology treatment would be given at weekly intervals at the start of a course of treatment. It is usually recommended that a client have a course of three to four treatments at regular weekly intervals when first having reflexology for a specific condition. After this time, there should be some improvement with the condition either cleared or improved, and it might be that from then on treatment is given at less frequent intervals to maintain the improvement. This would be particularly beneficial if the condition had been present for some time or the factors contributing to the condition are still present. The interval between treatments to maintain the improvement might be gradually extended to fortnightly, then three weekly, then monthly or six weekly, and a client will usually find an optimum time interval which is of most benefit to them. If regular treatments have been given and there is no improvement after three to four sessions, then it may be that reflexology is not going to be of benefit to the client at this time. In acute cases, such as a back or knee problem, it might be appropriate to give treatment twice weekly initially, provided the client is otherwise healthy. It is probably not advisable to give treatment too frequently, though, as the body needs time to adjust and for imbalances to be corrected. Most problems develop over a period of time, so it is unrealistic to expect these problems to be instantly corrected.

Chapter 6

Common Conditions That Can Be Treated

A wide range of conditions can be treated using reflexology. This is not to claim that reflexology is a miracle 'cure all', but there are very few conditions where it is not possible to give some benefit to the client even through clearing the condition, easing the condition or maintaining the condition. In nearly all cases, a person receiving reflexology will be relaxed after treatment, which will be extremely beneficial especially as so many conditions may be linked to stress.

In this chapter, when considering the approach to treatment for different conditions, this is looked at in terms of body systems and the more common conditions that might affect that system. For each body system there is a brief description of the parts making up this system and their function. A diagram shows the position of the reflex areas to these parts in the hands. For the conditions, the important reflex areas to treat for these conditions are mentioned.

To obtain the best results from treatment it is always best to give a full treatment by working all of the reflex areas found in both hands following the recommended order of treatment discussed in Chapter 5. In different conditions, different reflex areas are of greater importance to help ease the condition either by being the part directly affected (DR) or being areas that may be associated with the condition (AR). Extra attention will be given to these reflexes after working all of the reflexes in each hand, but before the solar plexus breathing exercise. The reflex areas requiring extra attention will be mentioned in connection with each condition and there will be a brief explanation as to why the named reflex areas might be helpful.

The musculoskeletal system

The skeletal system forms the bony framework of the body and can be divided into the axial skeleton (the skull, the vertebral column, the ribs and the sternum) and the appendicular skeleton (the upper limb: the shoulder girdle and the arm; the lower limb: the pelvic girdle and the leg). The main functions of the skeletal system are protection of the vital organs, a point of attachment for muscles, storage and release of minerals (calcium and phosphorus) and production of blood cells (in the bone marrow). The vertebral column (spine) can be divided into five regions: cervical, thoracic, lumbar, sacral and coccygeal; the upper limb includes the joints to the shoulder, elbow and wrist; the lower limb includes the joints to the hip, knee and ankle.

The muscular system includes three main types of muscle: skeletal (voluntary, striated), smooth (involuntary, non-striated) and cardiac (heart). By being able to contract and relax, muscles can produce movement of, for example, the skeleton (skeletal muscle) and internal organs such as the bladder, blood vessels, intestines (smooth muscle) and heart (cardiac muscle).

Arthritis

Arthritis involves pain and inflammation of a joint. There are many different forms of arthritis including osteoarthritis, rheumatoid arthritis and gout, but from the reflexology angle the approach to treatment is similar. The joints most commonly affected are the hips, knees, spine and fingers, with the joints becoming swollen, painful and having restricted movement. With gout it is often the big-toe joint that is affected and in this condition there is a build-up of uric acid in the blood due to overproduction or defective excretion by the kidneys, with sodium urate crystals being deposited in the joints and tendons. The affected joint will be painful, shiny, swollen and red.

DR: area affected e.g. hip, knee, spine

AR: areas nearby (e.g. lower spine, sacro-iliac joint, knee if hip is affected), adrenals (for inflammation), kidneys, large intestine, liver (for elimination), zone-related areas (e.g. elbow for knee)

The musculoskeletal system (PALMS OF THE HANDS)

LEFT

RIGHT

HEAD / BRAIN / SINUSES

HEAD / BRAIN / SINUSES

EUSTACHIAN TUBE
EYE
HEART
SOLAR PLEXUS
LYMPH DRAINAGE
TOP OF HEAD / BRAIN
PITUITARY
SIDE OF HEAD / BRAIN
PARATHYROIDS
NECK
THYROID
STOMACH / PANCREAS
ADRENAL
KIDNEY
URETER TUBE
BLADDER
RECTUM
SCIATIC

EUSTACHIAN TUBE
EYE
LUNG
LYMPH DRAINAGE
SIDE OF HEAD / BRAIN
TOP OF HEAD / BRAIN
PITUITARY
ADRENAL
KIDNEY
PARATHYROIDS
NECK
THYROID
STOMACH / PANCREAS
GALL BLADDER
URETER TUBE
BLADDER
SCIATIC

EARS
SHOULDER
SPLEEN
LIVER
TRANSVERSE COLON
WAIST LEVEL
DESCENDING COLON
ASCENDING COLON
SMALL INTESTINE
ILEO-CAECAL VALUE
SIGMOID COLON

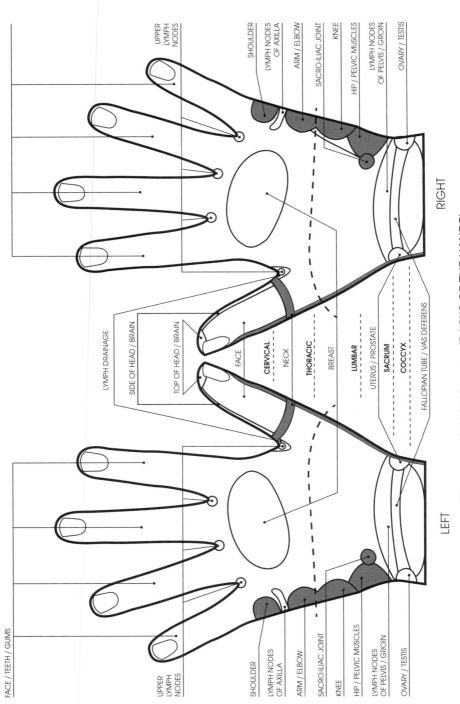

The musculoskeletal system (BACKS OF THE HANDS)

FACE / TEETH / GUMS

UPPER LYMPH NODES

SHOULDER
LYMPH NODES OF AXILLA
ARM / ELBOW
SACRO-ILIAC JOINT
KNEE
HIP / PELVIC MUSCLES
LYMPH NODES OF PELVIS / GROIN
OVARY / TESTIS

LEFT

LYMPH DRAINAGE
SIDE OF HEAD / BRAIN
TOP OF HEAD / BRAIN
FACE

CERVICAL
NECK

THORACIC
BREAST

LUMBAR
UTERUS / PROSTATE

SACRUM

COCCYX

FALLOPIAN TUBE / VAS DEFERENS

UPPER LYMPH NODES

SHOULDER
LYMPH NODES OF AXILLA
ARM / ELBOW
SACRO-ILIAC JOINT
KNEE
HIP / PELVIC MUSCLES
LYMPH NODES OF PELVIS / GROIN
OVARY / TESTIS

RIGHT

If a joint on one side is affected, then extra attention would also be given to the reflex area for the joint on the other side, as it may be compensating and perhaps is being overused, and when arthritis is present in one joint there is always the possibility that other joints may become affected.

Back (spine) problems

Back (spine) problems may involve such things as a pulled muscle, a strained ligament or a slipped (intervertebral) disc, and although it is not possible to diagnose the exact problem with reflexology, it is possible to treat these various problems. However, should a medical diagnosis not have been made and a person has had two or three reflexology treatments without improvement, then it is important that the patient be referred to a person who can make a diagnosis of the problem. Back problems are so common that often when working the reflex area to the spine it will appear tender, and on questioning the patient, it will be found that from time to time they suffer from a back problem. Treatment can help to strengthen this area and prevent frequent back problems. The most common regions affected are the cervical region (neck problems) and the lumbar region (lower backache, lumbago). Another consideration with a back problem is that the spinal nerves from the affected region may be involved and the nerve supply to areas of the body may be affected, causing problems with correct functioning of these areas. Neck problems may lead to shoulder and arm problems, and lower back problems may lead to problems in the leg such as sciatica.

DR: spine

AR: neck, shoulders, arms, elbows (if upper back problem), hips, knees, sacro-iliac joints, pelvic muscles, sciatic nerves (if lower back problem)

Bursitis

Bursitis is inflammation and swelling of a bursa, which is a fluid-filled sac that can form beneath the skin, usually over a joint, and which acts as a cushion between tendons and bones. A bursa can become inflamed due to injury or repetitive movement, and the common sites for a bursa to become inflamed are the shoulder, elbow, knee (housemaid's knee) and hip.

DR: area affected (e.g. shoulder, elbow, knee, hip)

AR: areas nearby (e.g. arm, elbow with shoulder problem), spine (for nerve supply), adrenals (for inflammation), zone-related areas (e.g. elbow for knee)

Carpal tunnel syndrome

Carpal tunnel syndrome is a wrist problem whereby the nerves entering the wrist through a fibrous band, called the carpal tunnel, at the joint become compressed causing tingling, numbness and pain in part of the hand (usually the thumb, index finger and middle finger as the median nerve is involved).

DR: arm

AR: elbow, shoulder, neck (all nearby areas), cervical spine (for nerve supply), adrenals (for inflammation), knee (for ankle, zone-related area)

Cramp

With cramp there is an involuntary contraction of a muscle or groups of muscles causing pain usually as a result of fatigue in the muscle or strain of the muscle. It is a problem that can affect a large number of people at night when cramp develops in the lower leg or foot.

DR: area affected (e.g. knee for lower leg)

AR: parathyroids, thyroid (for calcium balance), adrenals (for muscle tone), zone-related area (e.g. arm for leg)

Elbow problems (tennis elbow, golfer's elbow)

With tennis elbow there is inflammation of the outer side of the elbow; with golfers elbow there is inflammation of the inner side of the elbow. This condition need not necessarily occur from playing tennis or golf and can be caused by a variety of activities including gardening, painting, playing the violin and jobs that involve repeated use of the muscles and tendons of the forearm.

DR: elbow

AR: arm, shoulder, neck (areas nearby), cervical spine (for nerve supply), adrenals (for inflammation), knee (zone-related area)

Fibromyalgia

In fibromyalgia there is widespread musculoskeletal pain involving the muscles, tendons and ligaments. As well as a feeling of aching all over, there may be general fatigue, sleep disorder, headaches, irritable bowel syndrome (IBS) and multiple chemical sensitivity syndrome (to such things as odours, noise, bright lights, foods)

DR: areas affected (e.g. knee, hip for legs)

AR: pituitary, head/brain (if headaches), small intestine, large intestine (if IBS), adrenals (for inflammation, allergy)

Knee problems

Knee problems may involve the ligaments of the knee or the cartilages of the knee. Problems can develop from overuse, and the knee is a common site of injury in athletes.

DR: knee

AR: hips (areas nearby), lower spine (for nerve supply to leg), adrenals (for inflammation), elbow (zone-related areas)

Polymyalgia rheumatica

In polymyalgia rheumatica, the main symptom is one of stiffness in the muscles in the morning together with extreme tiredness, fever and sweating, loss of appetite, weight loss and depression. It is sometimes difficult to diagnose as symptoms are similar to many other conditions such as rheumatoid arthritis. The cause is unknown but may be genetic or linked to environmental factors.

DR: areas affected (e.g. arm, knee and hip for legs)

AR: spine (for nerve supply), head/brain (for depression), adrenals (for muscle tone, inflammation, stress)

Repetitive strain injury

A repetitive strain injury is one caused by repetitive use of an area, but the term 'repetitive strain injury' is often used to refer to problems involving the wrist joint. A common cause of this injury is from using a computer keyboard or mouse.

DR: arm and elbow

AR: neck, cervical spine (for nerve supply), shoulder (nearby area), adrenals (for inflammation), zone-related area (e.g. knee for ankle if wrist is affected)

Shoulder problems

Problems with the shoulder often result from a problem in the neck or upper spine. Common shoulder problems in women result from carrying bags on their shoulder or carrying children. Another common problem with the shoulder is a frozen shoulder where the joint becomes very painful and has restricted movement. Treatment may be helpful whether the problem is associated with the muscles or the ligaments of the shoulder joint.

DR: shoulder

AR: arm, elbow (nearby areas), neck, cervical spine, thoracic (for nerve supply), adrenals (for inflammation), hip (zone-related area)

Tendonitis

Tendons are the strong bands of tissue that attach muscle to bone and which help move the bones at a joint when the muscles contract. Tendonitis is inflammation of a tendon which may be caused by repetitive movements (e.g. using a computer keyboard or mouse) resulting in a repetitive strain injury (as above) or may be caused by a sudden awkward movement (e.g. throwing) or repeated overuse (e.g.

running). Common sites to be affected are the wrist and the ankle (Achilles tendon).

DR: area affected (e.g. arm for wrist, shoulder, knee for ankle)

AR: spine (for nerve supply to affect area), adrenals (for inflammation), zone-related area (e.g. knee, ankle for wrist)

The endocrine and reproductive systems

The endocrine or hormonal system includes the pituitary gland, thyroid gland, four parathyroid glands, pancreas, pineal gland and two adrenal glands. The secretions from the endocrine glands are called hormones and these help regulate the internal environment of the body. The reproductive system in the female includes the two ovaries, two fallopian (uterine) tubes, uterus, vulva and breasts (mammary glands). The reproductive system in the male includes the two testes, two epididymides, two spermatic cords, two vas deferens, two seminal vesicles, two ejaculatory ducts, prostate gland and penis.

Adrenal disorders
ADDISON'S DISEASE

In Addison's disease, the adrenal cortex fails to produce enough of its hormones. It is thought that most cases are due to an autoimmune condition that attacks the adrenal cortex, but it may also be due to damage to the adrenal cortex by, for example, surgery, cancer or degeneration of tissue. It may also be caused by a lack of adrenocorticotrophic hormone (ACTH) from the pituitary gland, which stimulates the adrenal cortex to produce its hormones. Symptoms may include weakness, fatigue and a tendency to become faint when getting out of bed or from a chair, and there may be increased pigmentation of the skin.

DR: adrenals

AR: pituitary (for adrenal control), thyroid, ovaries/testes (for hormonal balance), lymphatics, spleen (if an autoimmune condition)

CUSHING'S SYNDROME

In Cushing's syndrome, there is increased activity of the adrenal cortex due to an overproduction of ACTH. This produces symptoms of thin limbs, a fat trunk and rounded face, excessive hairiness with possible diabetes and high blood pressure.

DR: adrenals

AR: pituitary (for adrenal control), thyroid, ovaries/testes (for hormonal balance), heart, kidneys (for blood pressure), pancreas, liver, lymphatics (for diabetes)

The adrenals also produce hormones that have anti-inflammatory, anti-stress and anti-allergy actions, so they are very important in any condition when inflammation, stress or allergy is present. This is the case for nearly all conditions, so the adrenal gland reflex areas are possibly the most important in reflexology treatment.

Pancreas disorders
DIABETES MELLITUS

In the condition of diabetes mellitus, there is a deficiency of the hormone insulin usually caused by the pancreas not producing sufficient insulin. As the disorder progresses, other parts of the body can be affected by diabetes, especially the eyes (failing eyesight), kidneys (kidney failure), blood circulation (poor circulation) and lymphatic system (a reduced ability to fight infection). Particular care must be taken if a diabetic is taking insulin since reflexology treatment may encourage the pancreas to produce more insulin, in which case the medication being taken would need to be adjusted.

DR: pancreas

AR: liver, adrenals (both involved in carbohydrate metabolism), eyes, kidneys, heart, lymphatics (all may be affected)

Parathyroid disorders

Parathyroid gland problems are quite rare and caused by the glands producing too little (hypo) or too much (hyper) parathyroid hormone.

The endocrine and reproductive systems (PALMS OF THE HANDS)

LEFT

RIGHT

HEAD / BRAIN / SINUSES

EUSTACHIAN TUBE
EYE
HEART
SOLAR PLEXUS
LYMPH DRAINAGE
TOP OF HEAD / BRAIN
PITUITARY
SIDE OF HEAD / BRAIN
PARATHYROIDS
NECK
THYROID
STOMACH / PANCREAS
ADRENAL
KIDNEY
URETER TUBE
BLADDER
RECTUM
SCIATIC

EARS
SHOULDER
SPLEEN   LIVER
TRANSVERSE COLON
WAIST LEVEL
DESCENDING   ASCENDING
COLON   COLON
SMALL INTESTINE
ILEO-CAECAL VALUE
SIGMOID COLON

HEAD / BRAIN / SINUSES

EUSTACHIAN TUBE
EYE
LUNG
LYMPH DRAINAGE
SIDE OF HEAD / BRAIN
TOP OF HEAD / BRAIN
PITUITARY
ADRENAL
KIDNEY
PARATHYROIDS
NECK
THYROID
STOMACH / PANCREAS
GALL BLADDER
URETER TUBE
BLADDER
SCIATIC

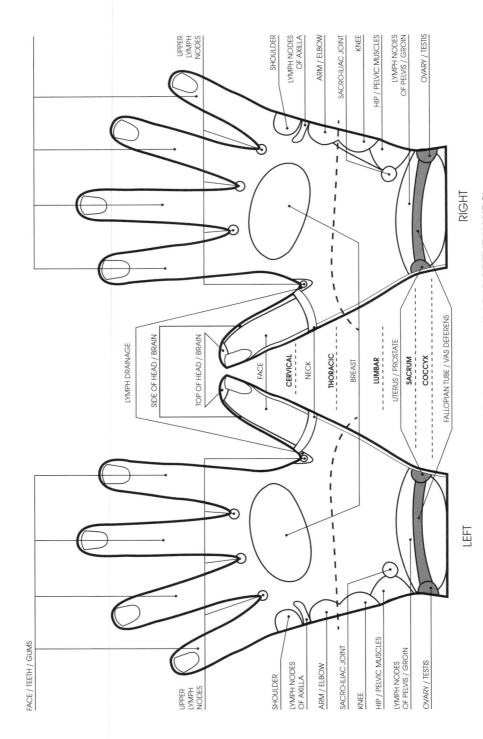

FACE / TEETH / GUMS

UPPER LYMPH NODES

SHOULDER
LYMPH NODES OF AXILLA
ARM / ELBOW
SACRO-ILIAC JOINT
KNEE
HIP / PELVIC MUSCLES
LYMPH NODES OF PELVIS / GROIN
OVARY / TESTIS

LYMPH DRAINAGE
SIDE OF HEAD / BRAIN
TOP OF HEAD / BRAIN
FACE
CERVICAL
NECK
THORACIC
BREAST
LUMBAR
UTERUS / PROSTATE
SACRUM
COCCYX
FALLOPIAN TUBE / VAS DEFERENS

UPPER LYMPH NODES

SHOULDER
LYMPH NODES OF AXILLA
ARM / ELBOW
SACRO-ILIAC JOINT
KNEE
HIP / PELVIC MUSCLES
LYMPH NODES OF PELVIS / GROIN
OVARY / TESTIS

LEFT

RIGHT

The endocrine and reproductive systems (BACKS OF THE HANDS)

HYPOPARATHYROIDISM

In hypoparathyroidism there is under-production of parathyroid hormone (PTH), which leads to a fall in blood calcium levels. It may occur following neck surgery. Symptoms may include a tingling sensation in the hands, feet or around the mouth, with muscle twitching, muscle spasms and muscle cramps. There may also be tiredness, irritability and depression.

DR: parathyroids

AR: thyroid (for calcium balance), adrenals (for muscle tone), head/brain (for depression)

HYPERPARATHYROIDISM

In hyperparathyroidism there is over-production of PTH which leads to a rise in blood calcium levels. Symptoms may include depression, tiredness, thirst, increased urination, nausea, constipation and muscle weakness, and long term there may be an increased risk of conditions such as osteoporosis, kidney stones, peptic ulcers and pancreatitis.

DR: parathyroids

AR: thyroid (for calcium balance), adrenals (for muscle tone), head/brain (for depression), kidneys, large intestine, stomach, pancreas (if affected)

Pineal disorders

SEASONAL AFFECTIVE DISORDER

Seasonal affective disorder is a type of depression that tends to occur during the winter months when the days are shorter and there is a reduced exposure to sunlight. The main symptoms are a low mood and lack of interest in everyday life. It is thought that the lack of sunlight reduces hypothalamus activity affecting production of the hormones melatonin and serotonin, plus affecting the body's internal clock.

DR: pituitary (for hypothalamus and pineal)

AR: adrenals (for stress), head/brain (for depression), solar plexus (for relaxation)

Pituitary disorders

Pituitary gland problems are quite uncommon and are usually caused by a tumour developing on the pituitary. Some of the more serious conditions would affect growth. If excess growth hormone is produced, the condition of *gigantism* will result, or *acromegaly* if this occurs after puberty. If there is a low level of growth hormone produced, the condition of *dwarfism* will result. Since the pituitary controls the activity of many of the other hormonal glands, any condition involving the pituitary may affect other hormonal glands.

DIABETES INSIPIDUS

In the condition of diabetes insipidus there is an excess production of antidiuretic hormone by the pituitary leading to an increased frequency to urinate, extreme thirst and an imbalance of electrolytes (high levels of sodium and potassium). This condition is quite rare.

DR: pituitary

AR: kidneys (parts affected)

Thyroid disorders
GOITRE

Goitre is an enlargement of the thyroid gland. It may be due to underactivity of the gland most probably due a deficiency of the mineral iodine needed for the formation of the thyroid hormones or over-activity of the gland with an excessive production of thyroxine.

DR: thyroid

AR: pituitary (for thyroid control), adrenals, ovaries or testes (for hormonal balance)

HYPERTHYROIDISM

In hyperthyroidism (thyrotoxicosis, overactivity of thyroid) there is excessive secretion of thyroxine such that metabolism is speeded up, and this can lead to weight loss even though the appetite is good, nervousness, anxiety, increased heart rate, palpitations, warm skin, sweating, diarrhoea, tremor and staring or protruding eyes.

DR: thyroid

AR: pituitary (for thyroid control), adrenals, ovaries or testes (for hormonal balance), heart, eyes, large intestine (all may be affected)

The thyroid gland can quite commonly be found to be imbalanced, becoming overactive or underactive. A similar approach to treatment is followed in both cases since treatment is working to restore balance of the thyroid gland.

HYPOTHYROIDISM

In hypothyroidism (myxoedema, underactivity of thyroid) there is a deficiency of the hormone thyroxine such that metabolism is slowed down, which can lead to a slow and sluggish mental state, weight gain though little appetite, the need for a lot of sleep but still feeling tired, thickening of the facial features so that the face becomes puffy, loss of body hair, constipation and low body temperature with the person feeling cold all the time.

DR: thyroid

AR: pituitary (for thyroid control), adrenals, ovaries or testes (for hormonal balance), heart, face, large intestine (all may be affected)

Female reproductive system

Breast lumps

Not all lumps in the breast are breast cancer, but any unusual changes to the breasts should always be checked. There are several different types of benign (non-cancerous) breast lumps that can occur, some of which are caused by hormonal changes that take place during the menstrual cycle.

DR: breast

AR: thoracic lymphatics (if infection or non-benign), adrenals (for inflammation), pituitary, thyroid, ovaries (for hormonal balance)

Cervicitis

Cervicitis refers to inflammation of the cervix which is usually associated with infection. It may be associated with high oestrogen levels in the blood or over-secretion of the glands in the cervix. Symptoms may include pain in the lower back, pelvis and legs, increased frequency of urination, painful menstruation and increased vaginal discharge (leukorrhoea).

DR: uterus

AR: ovaries, fallopian tubes (as parts of reproductive system), pituitary (for hormonal balance), pelvic lymphatics (for infection), adrenals (for inflammation), lower spine, hips, knees (for pain), kidneys, bladder (if affected)

Endometriosis

With endometriosis, endometrial tissue (the tissue that lines the uterus) is found in areas outside the uterus such as the ovaries and other parts of the pelvis. The endometrium is the lining of the womb that is usually shed at the time of a period in women, and the tissue found outside the uterus in this condition goes through the same process of thickening and shedding but cannot leave the body. It can lead to heavy and painful periods with pain in the lower abdomen, pelvis or lower back, and may also lead to fertility problems if the fallopian tubes and ovaries are damaged. There may also be depression and a lack of energy.

DR: parts affected (e.g. ovaries)

AR: uterus, fallopian tubes, ovaries (as parts of reproductive system), pituitary, thyroid, adrenals (for hormonal balance), spine (if back pain), head/brain (if depression)

Fibroid

A fibroid is a common, harmless tumour that can occur in or around the uterus. Fibroids can be quite small (the size of a pea) or quite large (the size of a melon). The presence of a fibroid will lead to heavy and painful menstruation, abdomen and lower back pain, an increased need to urinate, constipation and pain or discomfort during sex. Fibroids are thought to be linked to the hormone oestrogen.

DR: uterus

AR: ovaries, fallopian tubes (parts of reproductive system), pituitary, thyroid, adrenals (for hormonal balance), lower spine (if back pain), kidneys, bladder (if increased urination)

Infertility

Infertility refers to a failure to conceive and may be related to many factors including stress, hormone levels, a failure to ovulate, a blocked fallopian tube, endometriosis or fibroids. Problems with ovulation may be a result of conditions such as polycystic ovary syndrome, a thyroid problem or premature ovarian failure.

DR: ovaries

AR: uterus, fallopian tubes (as part of reproductive system), pituitary (for control of ovaries), thyroid (for hormonal balance), adrenals (for hormonal balance and stress), solar plexus (for relaxation)

Mastitis

With mastitis there is inflammation of the breast tissue with oedema and pain. The breast may also feel lumpy and there could be a discharge from the nipple. This condition most commonly occurs in women who are breastfeeding, though in some women it may occur prior to a period.

DR: breast

AR: adrenals (for inflammation), thoracic lymphatics (for infection)

Menopausal problems

Menopause refers to the time when the monthly periods in women end. The average age in the UK for menopause is 51 years, though some women may experience menopause in their 30s or 40s. The periods may suddenly stop or, more commonly, become less frequent with longer intervals between them before stopping completely. Menopause occurs due to a decrease in the levels of oestrogen produced, and a time known as the peri-menopause refers to the gradual decline building up to menopause. Many women experience problems at the time of peri-menopause and menopause, as the body has to adjust to the reduced levels of the female sex hormones. These problems can include symptoms such as hot flushes, depression, fatigue, migraines, digestive and urinary problems, and osteoporosis. Reflexology treatment does not prevent menopause but can help the body adjust to the hormonal changes. Often women follow a course of treatment as they approach menopause to try to prevent strong symptoms from developing. When symptoms are not relieved, a woman may require a hysterectomy (surgical removal of the uterus), and it may also involve removal of other associated areas such as the fallopian tubes and ovaries.

DR: ovaries, fallopian tubes, uterus

AR: pituitary, thyroid and parathyroids, adrenals (for hormonal balance), head/brain, large intestine, bladder (if these parts affected)

Menstrual problems

From the age of puberty to the time of menopause, a woman will have a monthly menstrual cycle where changes in the level of the female hormones produced by the ovaries cause changes in the parts of the female reproductive system in preparation to receive a fertilised ovum. If fertilisation does not occur, the lining of the uterus is shed at the time of menstruation together with some blood. Many women experience problems associated with the menstrual cycle, and these problems can often be helped by reflexology.

Amenorrhoea

Amenorrhoea (absence of periods) may refer to the periods never having started or when the periods have started and are then absent – when the first considerations must be pregnancy or the start of menopause. It may be due to hormonal imbalance, ovarian problems, or disorders of the thyroid or adrenal glands, and is often seen when there has been excessive weight loss due to an eating disorder or after stopping the contraceptive pill.

DR: ovaries, fallopian tubes, uterus

AR: pituitary, thyroid, adrenals (for hormonal balance), stomach (if eating disorder)

Dysmenorrhoea

Dysmenorrhoea, the pain associated with menstruation, may occur for a few days before a period starts or for the first few days of the period. As well as pain, there may be a feeling of bloating of the abdomen together with headaches or migraines, joint pains and nausea. It usually relates to a problem with the uterus.

DR: uterus

AR: ovaries, fallopian tubes (as parts of reproductive system), pituitary, thyroid, adrenals (for hormonal balance), abdominal lymphatics (for pain in abdomen), head/brain, eyes (for headaches and migraines), stomach (for nausea), knees, shoulders (if joint pain)

Metrorrhagia

Metrorrhagia (irregular periods) means that the menstrual cycle does not follow a regular pattern, with differing frequency of periods, differing amount of bleeding at the time of menstruation and differing length of time that menstruation lasts. It is usually associated with an imbalance of the hormones oestrogen and progesterone but can be affected by conditions such as polycystic ovary syndrome, extreme weight loss or excessive exercise, and also the contraceptive pill.

DR: ovaries

AR: uterus, fallopian tubes (as parts of reproductive system), pituitary, thyroid, adrenals (for hormonal balance)

Pre-menstrual syndrome

Over 150 different symptoms can be attributed to pre-menstrual syndrome, which is sometimes called pre-menstrual tension. The symptoms can occur for as long as 10 days prior to a period and can include mood changes, anxiety, irritability, lack of concentration, migraines, backache, breast discomfort, abdominal distension, fluid retention and constipation.

DR: ovaries, fallopian tubes, uterus

AR: pituitary, thyroid, adrenals (for hormonal balance), head/brain (for anxiety, mood changes), spine (for nerve supply and pain), abdominal lymphatics (for abdominal pain), kidneys (for fluid retention), large intestine (for constipation)

Ovarian cysts

A cyst is a fluid-filled sac, and it is not uncommon for cysts to form on the ovary where they are generally harmless and will just disappear. Symptoms may result if a cyst ruptures, as there will be pain in the pelvis, difficulty with emptying bowels and urinating, an alteration to the menstrual cycle, bloating of the abdomen and a possible effect on fertility.

DR: ovaries

AR: fallopian tubes, uterus (associated areas), pituitary (for hormonal balance), large intestine, kidneys (if affected), abdominal lymphatics (for bloating and pain)

Polycystic ovary syndrome

With polycystic ovary syndrome (PCOS) a number of cysts develop in the ovaries. These cysts are underdeveloped sacs in which the eggs develop but are unable to be released, meaning that ovulation cannot take place. Symptoms of PCOS may include irregular periods or no periods, difficulty in getting pregnant, excessive hair growth (on face, chest, back, buttocks), weight gain, thinning hair and acne. There is also an associated high level of insulin, which may lead to diabetes, and an increased production of the male hormone testosterone.

DR: ovaries

AR: pituitary, adrenals, thyroid (for hormonal balance), pancreas (for insulin control)

Salpingitis

With salpingitis there is inflammation of the fallopian tubes, and the infection may well have spread to this area from the uterus and could then spread to the ovaries. The condition may lead to blocked fallopian tubes, infertility and adhesions in the pelvis.

DR: fallopian tubes

AR: uterus, ovaries (as nearby parts), pelvic lymphatics (for infection), adrenals (for inflammation)

Vaginitis

With vaginitis there is inflammation of the vagina which may cause pain in the area and irritation. There may be an abnormal vaginal discharge and pain whilst urinating or having sex, and there may also be light bleeding or spotting. It can be caused by a number of infections including thrush, chlamydia or genital herpes, or it can be caused by irritants such as soap, washing powder or bath oil.

DR: uterus (includes area for vagina)

AR: pelvis lymphatics (for infection), adrenals (for inflammation)

Male reproductive system

Epididymitis

The epididymis is a tightly coiled mass of tubes that carries sperm from the testis to the vas deferens. The sperm mature as they pass through the epididymis and can be stored there temporarily. With epididymitis, symptoms may include pain in the testes, a swollen and red scrotum, painful urination and more frequent urination, painful intercourse, pain in the pelvis and enlarged lymph nodes in the groin.

DR: testes

AR: pelvic lymphatics (for infection), adrenals (for inflammation), kidneys, bladder (for problems with urination)

Erectile dysfunction

Erectile dysfunction (impotence) describes an inability of a man to achieve and maintain an erection of the penis. This can have many causes both psychological and physical (e.g. high blood pressure, heart disease, diabetes, scleroderma, kidney failure, cirrhosis of the liver).

DR: testes

AR: vas deferens, prostate (as parts of reproductive system), pituitary, thyroid (for hormonal balance), adrenals (for hormonal balance, inflammation, stress), heart, kidneys, liver (if affected), solar plexus (relaxation)

Infertility

Infertility in men may be caused by a number of problems including impotence (erectile dysfunction), sterility, low sperm count, decreased sperm mobility, abnormal sperm, low testosterone levels and premature ejaculation.

DR: testes

AR: vas deferens, prostate (as parts of reproductive system), pituitary, thyroid (for hormonal balance), adrenals (for hormonal balance, inflammation, stress), solar plexus (relaxation)

Orchitis

With orchitis there is inflammation of the testis and there may be pain in the testis, redness and swelling. There may also be fever, tiredness, headaches, general body aches and pain on urination.

DR: testes

AR: vas deferens, prostate (as parts of reproductive system), pelvic lymphatics (for infection), adrenals (for inflammation), head/brain (if headaches), kidneys, bladder (if problems with urination)

Prostate enlargement

Prostate enlargement occurs as men get older and because of the position of the prostate gland. As it enlarges it presses up on the bladder giving the impression of a greater sense of fullness in the bladder and therefore an increased need to empty the bladder. This problem can be particularly troublesome at night causing men to have interrupted sleep. Reflexology may help to alleviate the problem and reduce the need to empty the bladder so frequently.

DR: prostate

AR: bladder, ureter tubes, kidneys (for urinary system), adrenals (for inflammation), pelvic lymphatics (for infection)

Nervous system

The nervous system has two main divisions: the central nervous system and the peripheral nervous system. The central nervous system comprises the brain and the spinal cord; the peripheral nervous system comprises the 31 pairs of spinal nerves, 12 pairs of cranial nerves and the autonomic nervous system (sympathetic and parasympathetic systems).

The nervous system co-ordinates the activities of the other body systems so that the body functions smoothly. It is also the body's link with the outside world via the sense organs. It can detect changes within or outside the body (stimuli) and respond to them.

Bell's palsy

In Bell's palsy there is compression of the facial nerve (cranial nerve VII) which can lead to paralysis of the facial muscles. It is possibly caused by a virus or may occur following exposure to the cold.

DR: face

AR: head/brain (for cranial nerve), adrenals (for inflammation), lymphatics (for infection)

Dementia

Dementia (Alzheimer's disease) is a general term used to describe a loss of memory and other mental abilities, a loss which is severe enough to interfere with daily life. Alzheimer's disease is the most common type of dementia, and early symptoms may include difficulty in remembering recent conversations, names or events together with depression. As the condition deteriorates there may be impaired communication, poor judgement, disorientation, confusion, behaviour changes and difficulty with speaking, swallowing and walking.

DR: head/brain

AR: spine (nerve supply), hips, knees (if walking is affected), face, throat (if speech and swallowing are affected), solar plexus (relaxation), adrenals (stress), liver (for elimination)

Depression

Many people have times of feeling down, but with depression this feeling will last for weeks or months rather than just days. Depression affects people in different ways and there can be many different causes. There may be feelings of sadness, loss of interest in things, feeling tearful and feeling anxious, and there may also be physical symptoms such are tiredness, sleep problems, loss of appetite and various aches and pains. The severity of depression also varies from feeling persistently a bit low to feeling suicidal. Whilst it is advisable to seek medical help for depression, reflexology may be of help in addition to medical treatment offered.

DR: head/brain

AR: adrenals (for stress), spine (for nerve supply), solar plexus (for relaxation), liver (for elimination of toxins)

The nervous system (PALMS OF THE HANDS)

LEFT   RIGHT

HEAD / BRAIN / SINUSES

EUSTACHIAN TUBE
EYE
HEART
SOLAR PLEXUS
LYMPH DRAINAGE
TOP OF HEAD / BRAIN
PITUITARY
SIDE OF HEAD / BRAIN
PARATHYROIDS
NECK
THYROID
STOMACH / PANCREAS
ADRENAL
KIDNEY
URETER TUBE
BLADDER
RECTUM
SCIATIC

EARS
SHOULDER
SPLEEN   LIVER
TRANSVERSE COLON
WAIST LEVEL
DESCENDING   ASCENDING
COLON   COLON
SMALL INTESTINE
ILEO-CAECAL VALUE
SIGMOID COLON

HEAD / BRAIN / SINUSES

EUSTACHIAN TUBE
EYE
LUNG
LYMPH DRAINAGE
SIDE OF HEAD / BRAIN
TOP OF HEAD / BRAIN
PITUITARY
ADRENAL
KIDNEY
PARATHYROIDS
NECK
THYROID
STOMACH / PANCREAS
GALL BLADDER
URETER TUBE
BLADDER
SCIATIC

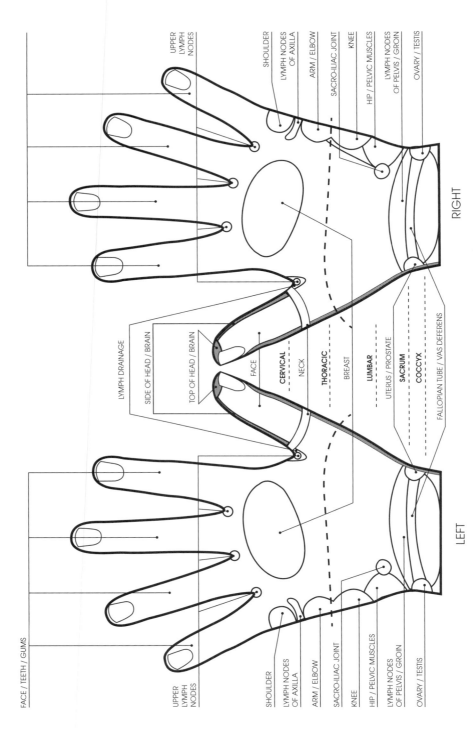

FACE / TEETH / GUMS

UPPER LYMPH NODES

SHOULDER

LYMPH NODES OF AXILLA

ARM / ELBOW

SACRO-ILIAC JOINT

KNEE

HIP / PELVIC MUSCLES

LYMPH NODES OF PELVIS / GROIN

OVARY / TESTIS

LEFT

LYMPH DRAINAGE

SIDE OF HEAD / BRAIN

TOP OF HEAD / BRAIN

FACE

CERVICAL

NECK

THORACIC

BREAST

LUMBAR

UTERUS / PROSTATE

SACRUM

COCCYX

FALLOPIAN TUBE / VAS DEFERENS

UPPER LYMPH NODES

SHOULDER

LYMPH NODES OF AXILLA

ARM / ELBOW

SACRO-ILIAC JOINT

KNEE

HIP / PELVIC MUSCLES

LYMPH NODES OF PELVIS / GROIN

OVARY / TESTIS

RIGHT

The nervous system (BACKS OF THE HANDS)

Ear problems
EARACHE AND EAR INFECTIONS

Earache and ear infections are common, and pain felt in the ear is usually due to infection particularly involving the middle ear. Any infection must be treated quickly in order that the infection does not spread to the inner ear and affect hearing or balance. Those with a tendency towards ear infections can work the reflex areas to try to prevent these frequent infections.

DR: ears, Eustachian tubes

AR: upper lymphatics (for infection), side of head/brain (for nerve supply), solar plexus (for relaxation), adrenals (to reduce inflammation)

DEAFNESS

Deafness may be due to a number of factors, and with age the hearing often does deteriorate. A simple problem causing deafness may be wax in the ear which is blocking the pathway down to the eardrum and thus affecting normal hearing. Other problems can include damage to the eardrum or to the middle ear, including blocked Eustachian tubes as may be caused by a cold or by 'glue ear' (whereby mucus builds up in the middle ear). Deafness can also involve the hearing receptors in the inner ear or the hearing areas of the brain.

DR: ears, Eustachian tubes

AR: side of head/brain, neck, cervical spine (for nerve supply), solar plexus (for relaxation), adrenals (for inflammation, stress), upper lymphatics (for infection)

TINNITUS

With tinnitus, a person experiences noises in the ear. The noise may be a persistent ringing, buzzing or humming, and often becomes more noticeable when it is quiet and therefore makes it difficult for a person with tinnitus to relax or go off to sleep.

DR: ears, Eustachian tubes

AR: side of head/brain (for nerve supply), neck, cervical spine (for nerve supply), solar plexus (for relaxation), adrenals (for inflammation and stress)

VERTIGO

With vertigo, the balance mechanism of the inner ear is affected. A person will think that stationary objects around them are moving and may then feel dizzy, lose their balance and may fall.

DR: ears

AR: Eustachian tubes (as part of ears), side of head/brain (for nerve supply), neck, cervical spine (for nerve supply), eyes, solar plexus (for relaxation), adrenals (for inflammation and stress)

EPILEPSY

With epilepsy, there are episodes of excessive activity in a part of the brain, causing fits. The severity of the seizures vary from person to person with some experiencing a short loss of awareness or just an odd feeling while others may lose consciousness and have convulsions. For some, the condition may be genetic, whilst in others it may be caused by a severe head injury, stroke or brain tumour.

DR: head/brain

AR: adrenals (for stress), solar plexus (relaxation)

Eye problems
IMPAIRED VISION

Many people suffer from eyesight problems, and although reflexology may not reverse this problem, it may help to prevent deterioration of the eyesight. By working the eye reflex, the muscles of the eye are stimulated to work more efficiently if they have become lazy, and the nerves to the eye are also treated to ensure good nerve supply.

DR: eyes

AR: neck, cervical spine (for nerve supply), head/brain (control of eye function), kidneys (zone related), adrenals (for inflammation, stress)

CONJUNCTIVITIS

Conjunctivitis is a common infection of the eye where the eye becomes red and itchy. It can also be caused by an allergic reaction. By rubbing the affected eye and then the other eye it is easy for the infection to spread to both eyes. Those with a tendency towards eye infections such as conjunctivitis can work the reflex areas to try to prevent these frequent infections.

DR: eyes

AR: upper lymphatics (for infection), adrenals (for inflammation)

DRY EYES

When the eyes are dry, insufficient tears are being produced. It is the tears that help to lubricate the eyes and remove dirt and dust which might irritate the eyes, so when the eyes become dry they become sore and itchy.

DR: eyes

AR: upper lymphatics (for infection), adrenals (for inflammation, allergy)

CATARACTS

A cataract affects the lens of the eye and causes the lens to lose its opacity which can lead to blurred or misty vision. As the cataract becomes worse, the sight deteriorates and eventually surgery will be required to remove and replace the affected lens. Cataract is common in the elderly and also diabetics.

DR: eyes

AR: head/brain (for eye function), kidneys (zone-related), pancreas (if diabetic)

GLAUCOMA

Glaucoma is a more serious eye problem whereby there is an increase in pressure within the eye (intraocular pressure) due to defective draining of the aqueous humour from the eye. Symptoms may include reduced vision (the peripheral or outer field of vision), painful eyes, seeing coloured haloes around lights and headaches. It occurs most commonly in the elderly.

DR: eyes

AR: neck (for nerve supply), head/brain (for eye function), kidneys (zone related)

HEADACHES AND MIGRAINES

Headaches are a common condition from which most people suffer at some time. A migraine involves a severe headache and may also be accompanied by visual disturbances and feelings of nausea. There can be many possible causes of headaches and migraines including allergy to certain foods or other substances, dietary factors such as too much fat in the diet, association with the menstrual cycle or menopause in women, neck and upper spine problems, sinus congestion, eye strain or constipation – leading to a build-up of toxins in the system, high blood pressure, tension and stress.

Often the patient is aware of the cause of the problem, but if not, it should be possible to determine the cause by finding out which reflex areas are the most tender in the hands. Migraine sufferers can be greatly helped by reflexology either totally clearing the condition or greatly reducing the frequency and severity of attacks.

DR: top of the head, side of the head

AR: neck, cervical spine (for nerve supply), ovaries (in women), pituitary (for hormonal balance), sinuses (if there is congestion), eyes (if affected), liver, large intestine, kidneys (for elimination), heart (for circulation), adrenals (for inflammation, stress, allergy), solar plexus (for relaxation)

INSOMNIA AND SLEEP PROBLEMS

Many people suffer from insomnia and sleep problems, and this may involve difficulty in getting to sleep or waking during the night and not being able to return to sleep. It can be due to stress and worry, depression, pain – such as arthritic pain, severe earache or menopause in women (hot flushes) – or may result from adjusting to time differences as with jet lag.

DR: pituitary/pineal, head/brain

AR: solar plexus (for relaxation), adrenals (for stress), spine, hip, knee, ear (if these areas are affected), pituitary, ovaries (for menopause)

MOTOR NEURONE DISEASE

With motor neurone disease there is a progressive degeneration of motor neurones in the brain and spinal cord, leading to symptoms of weakness and twitching of muscles, and then paralysis first in the hand, arms and shoulder girdle, and later affecting the legs. It occurs in men more frequently than women.

DR: head/brain, spine

AR: shoulders, arms, elbows, hips, knees, (if affected), adrenals (muscle tone)

MULTIPLE SCLEROSIS

With multiple sclerosis the transmission of the nerve impulses is affected and symptoms such as muscle weakness, loss of control of movements, loss of balance and loss of sensation in parts of the body may develop. Sometimes the eyes can be affected. There can be periods of remission when the symptoms disappear, but they return as the condition progresses. The exact cause is not known, though it may be caused by a virus.

DR: head/brain, neck, spine

AR: shoulder, arm, hip, knee, eye, bladder, large intestine (if area is affected), adrenals (for inflammation), lymphatics (for infection)

NEURALGIA

In neuralgia there is intense pain along a nerve, and this is most common in the head or face. Trigeminal neuralgia involves the trigeminal nerve (cranial nerve V) and causes pain in the face. Post-herpetic neuralgia can follow an attack of shingles and is a persistent nerve pain in the site that has been affected by shingles.

DR: face

AR: head/brain, spine (for nerve supply)

PARKINSON'S DISEASE

With Parkinson's disease there is damage to the nervous system controlling the muscles. This can lead to stiffness and weakness in the muscles with movement becoming uncoordinated. There may be symptoms of tremor – particularly noticeable in the hands, and walking may be affected – the person may shuffle their feet and a 'mask-like' look can develop due to the face muscles not functioning correctly.

DR: head/brain

AR: spine, neck (for nerve supply), adrenals (for inflammation), shoulders, arms, hips, knees, face, bladder, large intestine (if area affected)

SCIATICA

The sciatic nerve, which runs from the lower back down the back of the leg, can become inflamed and the condition of sciatica results, causing pain along any part of the region which the nerve supplies. Sciatica usually results from a problem with the lower spine or the pelvis.

DR: sciatic nerve

AR: lumbar and sacral spine (for nerve supply), sacro-iliac joint, muscles of the pelvis, hip, knee (if area affected), adrenals (for inflammation)

SHINGLES

In shingles (herpes zoster neuritis), the herpes zoster virus affects the posterior root ganglion of a nerve and then passes along the sensory nerve to the skin. The skin becomes inflamed and vesicles appear on the skin surface causing pain in the area and hypersensitivity. The most commonly affected areas are the upper body, but the cornea of the eye may be affected or the scalp.

DR: areas affected (e.g. top of head, arms)

AR: adrenals (for inflammation, stress), solar plexus (for relaxation), lymphatics (for infection)

STRESS

Stress (tension) is probably the most common condition experienced in modern times and can result in a range of different conditions such as migraines, insomnia, eczema, asthma or irritable bowel syndrome. The general relaxing effect of reflexology treatment, and the one-to-one contact with the practitioner for a whole hour when problems can be discussed, can be very beneficial to people suffering from stress. Although treatment may not be able to take away the reasons for the stress, which may be external factors such as family or work situations, often a person finds that they are able to cope with the stress better as a result of treatment.

DR: head/brain

AR: pituitary, adrenals (for stress), solar plexus (for relaxation) + to areas linked to physical symptoms (e.g. head, lungs, intestines)

STROKE

With a stroke or cerebral haemorrhage a blood clot develops in the cerebral region of the brain. The clot is usually on one side of the brain, and the result of a stroke is a partial or a total paralysis of the opposite side of the body to the side of the brain affected, since the right side of the brain controls the muscles of the left side of the body and the left side of the brain controls the muscles of the right side of the body. Speech may also be affected. Factors such as high blood pressure and poor circulation may lead to a stroke. Depending on the severity of the stroke, some patients make a better recovery than others. In general, the sooner a patient is treated after suffering a stroke, the better the results.

DR: head/brain

AR: neck, spine (for nerve supply), heart (for circulation), adrenals, shoulders, arms (if arms are affected), hips, knees (if legs are affected), face (if speech is affected)

With the more serious disorders of the nervous system such as stroke,   loss of control of the emptying of the bladder and constipation can respond very well to treatment. More obvious improvements can take time, though people often express a sense of feeling better in themselves and coping better with daily tasks. It may well be that treatment needs to be given over a considerable period of time, maybe months or years, to try to achieve improvement or to halt the deterioration of the condition.

Digestive system

The digestive system includes the mouth, teeth, pharynx, oesophagus, stomach, small intestine, large intestine, rectum and anus, plus the accessory glands (the liver, gall bladder and pancreas). The main function of the digestive system is to ingest food, break it down and absorb useful items and excrete unwanted material.

Problems in the mouth

TOOTHACHE

If there is persistent toothache, a visit to the dentist is required, but reflexology may be able to help relieve toothache. The pain may be due to infection around the teeth or a cavity in the tooth.

DR: teeth/gums, face

AR: upper   lymphatics   (for   infection),   adrenals   (for inflammation), solar plexus (relaxation)

MOUTH ULCERS

Mouth ulcers are sores on the gums which may result from poor mouth hygiene or from foods that are eaten that aggravate the gums.

DR: teeth and gums, face

AR: upper lymphatics (for infection), adrenals (for inflammation)

Stomach problems

GASTRITIS

With gastritis there is inflammation of the lining of the stomach when insufficient mucus is produced in the stomach to protect it against the acidic environment. There may be pain in the stomach, nausea and a loss of appetite. It may be caused by too much rich food and certain drugs (e.g. aspirin, excess alcohol), infection by bacteria or stress. In a chronic state, the condition of *pernicious anaemia* may result due to damage to the stomach cells producing intrinsic factor.

DR: stomach

AR: adrenals (for inflammation, stress), abdominal lymphatics (for infection)

HIATUS HERNIA

A hernia is an abnormal protrusion of internal body parts through a weakness in the surrounding muscles. With an hiatus hernia, the stomach pushes up through the gap (hiatus) in the diaphragm through which the oesophagus passes. The main symptom is heartburn, which will be worse after eating a large meal or from lying down or bending. It can be associated with obesity or pregnancy.

DR: stomach

AR: diaphragm, oesophagus (areas involved), adrenals (for inflammation), thoracic spine (nerve supply)

INDIGESTION

Indigestion (dyspepsia) is pain in the stomach region and is not only due to the types of foods eaten but how they are eaten. Often indigestion is linked to eating too quickly or in a stressed state.

DR: stomach

AR: oesophagus (area nearby), solar plexus (for relaxation), adrenals (for stress, allergy)

The digestive system (PALMS OF THE HANDS)

LEFT

RIGHT

HEAD / BRAIN / SINUSES

EUSTACHIAN TUBE
EYE
HEART
SOLAR PLEXUS
LYMPH DRAINAGE
TOP OF HEAD / BRAIN
PITUITARY
SIDE OF HEAD / BRAIN
PARATHYROIDS
NECK
THYROID
STOMACH / PANCREAS
ADRENAL
KIDNEY
URETER TUBE
BLADDER
RECTUM
SCIATIC

EARS
SHOULDER
SPLEEN
LIVER
TRANSVERSE COLON
WAIST LEVEL
DESCENDING COLON
ASCENDING COLON
SMALL INTESTINE
ILEO-CAECAL VALUE
SIGMOID COLON

HEAD / BRAIN / SINUSES

EUSTACHIAN TUBE
EYE
LUNG
LYMPH DRAINAGE
SIDE OF HEAD / BRAIN
TOP OF HEAD / BRAIN
PITUITARY
ADRENAL
KIDNEY
PARATHYROIDS
NECK
THYROID
STOMACH / PANCREAS
GALL BLADDER
URETER TUBE
BLADDER
SCIATIC

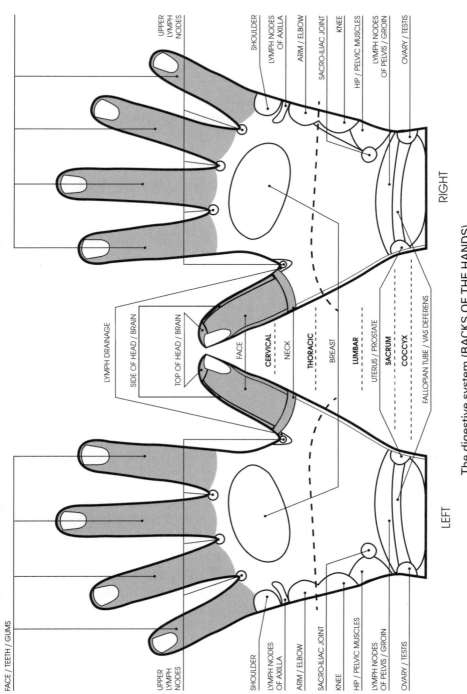

FACE / TEETH / GUMS

UPPER LYMPH NODES

SHOULDER

LYMPH NODES OF AXILLA

ARM / ELBOW

SACRO-ILIAC JOINT

KNEE

HIP / PELVIC MUSCLES

LYMPH NODES OF PELVIS / GROIN

OVARY / TESTIS

LYMPH DRAINAGE

SIDE OF HEAD / BRAIN

TOP OF HEAD / BRAIN

FACE

CERVICAL

NECK

THORACIC

BREAST

LUMBAR

UTERUS / PROSTATE

SACRUM

COCCYX

FALLOPIAN TUBE / VAS DEFERENS

UPPER LYMPH NODES

SHOULDER

LYMPH NODES OF AXILLA

ARM / ELBOW

SACRO-ILIAC JOINT

KNEE

HIP / PELVIC MUSCLES

LYMPH NODES OF PELVIS / GROIN

OVARY / TESTIS

RIGHT

LEFT

The digestive system (BACKS OF THE HANDS)

STOMACH ULCER

A stomach ulcer (gastric ulcer) is an open sore on the lining of the stomach. An ulcer can also occur in the duodenum (duodenal ulcer) and both these types of ulcers are sometimes known as peptic ulcers. When an ulcer is present there may be symptoms of pain in the stomach, indigestion, heartburn and nausea. They may be caused by a bacterial infection or from drugs such as aspirin, or ibuprofen used over a long time or in high doses.

DR: stomach

AR: diaphragm, oesophagus (areas nearby), adrenals (for inflammation), abdominal lymphatics (for infection)

Intestinal problems
COLITIS

Colitis refers to inflammation of the colon (large intestine), and one form of colitis is mucous colitis or irritable bowel syndrome. Another more serious form is ulcerative colitis whereby ulcers form in the walls of the large intestine. Symptoms include abdominal pain and diarrhoea with blood in the stools due to bleeding from the ulcers. In severe cases anaemia and dehydration can result.

DR: large intestine

AR: small intestine, adrenals (for inflammation), heart (for circulation)

CONSTIPATION

Constipation refers to irregular bowel movement and difficulty with emptying the bowel. It may be linked to lack of roughage in the diet, lack of fluid intake, poor muscle tone in the intestines or poor nerve supply to the intestines. Since the large intestine is an important eliminating organ, if elimination is not taking place then toxins are accumulating in the body and can lead to other conditions such as headaches, skin problems, sinus problems and circulatory problems.

DR: large intestine

AR: small intestine (area nearby), adrenals (for muscle tone, stress), solar plexus (for relaxation), lumbar spine (for nerve supply), head/brain (for headaches), sinuses (for sinus congestion), heart (for circulation), liver, kidneys (for elimination)

CROHN'S DISEASE

Crohn's disease is inflammation of the lining of the digestive system most commonly involving the small intestine (ileum) and large intestine (colon). It can cause symptoms of pain in the abdomen, diarrhoea, fatigue, weight loss, and blood and mucous in the stools. It may be a genetic condition or involve the immune system (autoimmune condition).

DR: small intestine, large intestine

AR: abdominal lymphatics (for infection), adrenals (for inflammation), lumbar spine (for nerve supply)

DIARRHOEA

Diarrhoea refers to increased frequency in emptying the bowels with a more fluid content to the stools. Short term it is the body's way of removing foods that it has found unsuitable, so it is not a problem, but long term there is the risk of dehydration since the undigested food is not long enough in the large intestine for water to be reabsorbed and also the food will have passed through the small intestine too quickly, so the correct breakdown and absorption of food will not have taken place. Diarrhoea accompanied by severe abdominal pain, especially on the left side, may be a symptom of *diverticulitis*.

DR: large intestine

AR: small intestine (area nearby), adrenals (for inflammation, allergy), lymphatics (for infection)

HAEMORRHOIDS

Haemorrhoids (piles) are varicose veins in the rectum often associated with overstraining due to constipation.

DR: rectum

AR: large intestine, small intestine, adrenals (for muscle tone), spine (for nerve supply), heart (for circulation)

IRRITABLE BOWEL SYNDROME

Irritable bowel syndrome (also known as mucous colitis) refers to a condition whereby the bowel is irritable. There is pain in the abdomen, constipation and then diarrhoea, and an excess of mucus in the stools. There may also be flatulence, distension in the abdomen and abdominal rumblings. The condition is thought to be stress related, though foods can also affect the condition.

DR: large intestine, small intestine

AR: adrenals (for inflammation, stress, allergy), solar plexus (for relaxation), spine (for nerve supply)

Liver disorders
CIRRHOSIS

With cirrhosis of the liver, there is scarring of liver tissue which prevents the liver from working properly. It usually results from long-term liver damage typically associated with drinking excess alcohol over many years or being infected with the hepatitis C virus. There may be few symptoms initially, but there may be loss of appetite, nausea and itchy skin, and in the later stages jaundice may develop and there may be very dark faeces, vomiting of blood, shortness of breath and oedema in the legs.

DR: liver

AR: lymphatics, spleen (if infection), adrenals (for inflammation), stomach, large intestine, lungs, knee (if affected)

HEPATITIS

With hepatitis, there is inflammation of the liver caused by a viral infection. It can also result from drinking excess alcohol over many years. Initial symptoms of hepatitis are similar to those of influenza with muscle and joint pains, high temperature, nausea, headache, plus there may be jaundice. The most common types of hepatitis are hepatitis A, hepatitis B and hepatitis C.

DR: liver

AR: lymphatics, spleen (for infection), adrenals (for inflammation), head/brain (for headaches), knees, hips, shoulders, arms (for muscle and joint pains), stomach (for nausea)

JAUNDICE

With jaundice, there is a build-up of bilirubin, a bile pigment, in the blood and tissues which causes them to turn yellow. This is particularly noticeable in the skin and the whites of the eyes. It may be due to bile not draining from the gall bladder as a result of gallstones or to disease of the liver. Jaundice can sometimes occur in newborn babies but usually clears within a few weeks.

DR: liver

AR: gall bladder (for bile drainage), lymphatics (for infection)

Gall bladder disorders
CHOLECYSTITIS

In the condition of cholecystitis there is inflammation of the gall bladder leading to a sudden sharp pain in the region of the gall bladder on the right side of the body, and the pain can spread upwards to the right shoulder. It may be caused by a blockage to the cystic duct, the opening into the gall bladder, and the blockage may be due to a gallstone or a mixture of bile and cholesterol. The blockage prevents bile from leaving the gall bladder, which then becomes inflamed.

DR: gall bladder

AR: liver (for bile production), adrenals (for inflammation), thoracic lymphatics (for infection)

GALLSTONES

Gallstones are supposedly more common in females who are 'fair, fat, fertile and flatulent'! These small stones that form in the gall bladder are usually made up of cholesterol and are often associated with a diet high in fats. If the stones are small, it may be possible to help them to be passed and they will pass down in the bile from the gall bladder to the small intestine and then be eliminated through the large intestine.

DR: gall bladder

AR: liver (for bile production), small intestine, large intestine (for elimination), adrenals (for inflammation)

Integumentary system

The integumentary system includes the skin together with the hair and nails. The main functions of the skin include protection, temperature control and excretion. There are also numerous sensory receptors in the skin that can detect pain, temperature, touch and pressure.

Acne

Acne is often associated with puberty and results in cysts forming on the skin, particularly on the face, chest and top of the back, and these can sometimes cause scarring of the skin. There is an increased secretion of sebum by the sebaceous glands which blocks the sebaceous ducts and hair follicles in the skin. As well as the effect of the hormone levels, dietary factors may be a cause.

DR:　face

AR:　adrenals (for inflammation, stress, allergy), ovaries or testes, pituitary (for hormonal balance), solar plexus (for relaxation), lymphatics (for infection), liver and gall bladder (for elimination)

Dermatitis

With dermatitis, there is inflammation of the skin due to allergy and the condition is very similar to eczema. An itchy rash develops on the skin and often the face, eyes, arms and elbows can be affected.

DR:　face, eyes, arms and elbows

AR:　adrenals (for inflammation, stress, allergy), solar plexus (for relaxation), lymphatics (for infection)

Eczema

With eczema, the skin is dry, flaky and itchy. It can often occur in babies and young children whereby it results from an allergy especially to cow's milk. Many youngsters grow out of the condition, but it can reoccur in adult life often linked to allergy, dietary factors and stress. The common sites for eczema are the face, ears as well as the arms and legs, particularly in the creases of the joints.

DR: face, ears, arms, legs

AR: adrenals (for inflammation, stress, allergy), solar plexus (for relaxation), lymphatics (for infection), large intestine, kidneys, liver (for elimination), heart (for circulation)

Psoriasis

With psoriasis, slightly raised red patches appear on the skin covered by silver scales which flake off leaving a red map-like rash on the skin. Common areas to be affected are the elbows, knees and scalp. Linked to the psoriasis, the nails are often pitted and ridged, and arthritis can develop in the joints.

DR: areas affected (e.g. top of head, arms, knees)

AR: adrenals (for inflammation, stress), solar plexus (for relaxation), lymphatics (for infection)

Urinary system

The urinary system is composed of the two kidneys, two ureter tubes, the bladder and the urethra. Its main functions are excretion of urine and maintenance of the fluid and electrolyte levels in the body. The urine is produced in the kidneys, then passes down the ureter tubes to the bladder where it is stored before being eliminated through the urethra.

Cystitis

Cystitis is inflammation and infection of the bladder. It causes an increased need to empty the bladder and often a burning sensation on urination. Those who suffer from cystitis may find that the condition reoccurs when they get tired and run down, and regular reflexology treatment may help to strengthen this area and the lymphatic system so that repeated infections do not occur.

DR: bladder

AR: ureter tubes, kidneys (parts of urinary system), pelvic lymphatics (for infection), adrenals (for inflammation)

Incontinence

Incontinence refers to an inability to control the emptying of the bladder and may be due to damage to the nerve supply to the bladder or involve weakness in the pelvic muscles. In children, bedwetting may occur due to emotional factors but the problem can still be helped sometimes.

DR: bladder

AR: ureter tubes, kidneys (parts of urinary system), pelvic lymphatics (for infection), adrenals (for inflammation), lumbar and sacral spine (for nerve supply)

Kidney stones

Stones can form in the kidney(s) and are often only about the size of a grape pip, though they can be larger. They are usually made up of calcium, and provided they are small, they may be passed from the kidney in the urine. As the stone passes down the ureter tube to the bladder, pain may be felt (renal colic).

DR: kidneys

AR: ureter tubes, bladder (part of urinary system), adrenals (for inflammation), thyroid and parathyroids (for calcium balance)

Oedema

Oedema refers to fluid retention in the body, and the build-up of fluid causes swelling of the affected part. This can occur almost anywhere in the body, but it is most common in the feet and ankles (peripheral oedema), though it might affect the brain, lungs or eyes. There can be many different causes, the most common being sitting or standing for long periods. However, it might also be associated with disease of the kidneys, heart, lungs, liver or thyroid, and with pregnancy.

DR: area affected (e.g. knee for lower leg)

AR: kidneys (for elimination), ureter tubes, bladder (as parts of urinary system), lymphatics (for fluid retention), heart, lungs, liver, thyroid (if affected)

Urethritis

Urethritis is inflammation of the urethra and is usually caused by an infection. There may be pain or a burning sensation on urination, and in men the tip of the penis may feel irritated and sore. In women the symptoms may be less noticeable, unless the infections spread to areas such as the uterus or fallopian tubes and causes pelvic inflammatory disease.

DR: bladder

AR: ureter tubes, kidneys (part of urinary system), pelvic lymphatics (for infection), adrenals (for inflammation), prostate, uterus, fallopian tubes (if affected)

HEAD / BRAIN / SINUSES

EUSTACHIAN TUBE
EYE
LUNG
LYMPH DRAINAGE
SIDE OF HEAD / BRAIN
TOP OF HEAD / BRAIN
PITUITARY
ADRENAL
KIDNEY
PARATHYROIDS
NECK
THYROID
STOMACH / PANCREAS
GALL BLADDER
URETER TUBE
BLADDER
SCIATIC

RIGHT

EARS
SHOULDER
SPLEEN   LIVER
TRANSVERSE COLON
WAIST LEVEL
DESCENDING COLON   ASCENDING COLON
SMALL INTESTINE
ILEO-CAECAL VALUE
SIGMOID COLON

LEFT

HEAD / BRAIN / SINUSES

EUSTACHIAN TUBE
EYE
HEART
SOLAR PLEXUS
LYMPH DRAINAGE
TOP OF HEAD / BRAIN
PITUITARY
SIDE OF HEAD / BRAIN
PARATHYROIDS
NECK
THYROID
STOMACH / PANCREAS
ADRENAL
KIDNEY
URETER TUBE
BLADDER
RECTUM
SCIATIC

The urinary system (PALMS OF THE HANDS)

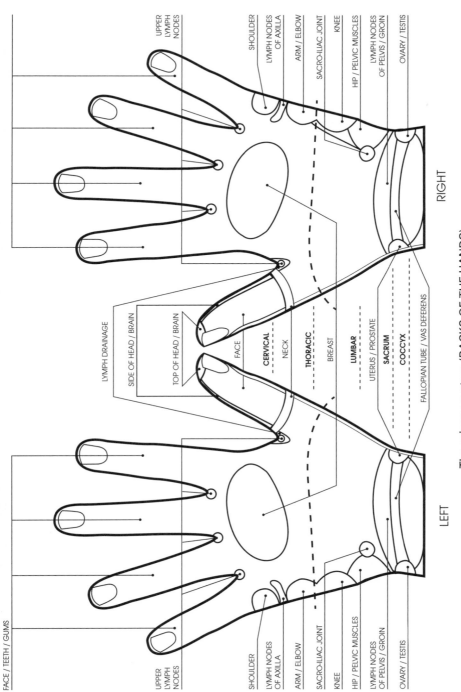

The urinary system (BACKS OF THE HANDS)

FACE / TEETH / GUMS

UPPER LYMPH NODES

SHOULDER
LYMPH NODES OF AXILLA
ARM / ELBOW
SACRO-ILIAC JOINT
KNEE
HIP / PELVIC MUSCLES
LYMPH NODES OF PELVIS / GROIN
OVARY / TESTIS

LEFT

RIGHT

LYMPH DRAINAGE
SIDE OF HEAD / BRAIN
TOP OF HEAD / BRAIN
FACE
CERVICAL
NECK
THORACIC
BREAST
LUMBAR
UTERUS / PROSTATE
SACRUM
COCCYX
FALLOPIAN TUBE / VAS DEFERENS

UPPER LYMPH NODES

SHOULDER
LYMPH NODES OF AXILLA
ARM / ELBOW
SACRO-ILIAC JOINT
KNEE
HIP / PELVIC MUSCLES
LYMPH NODES OF PELVIS / GROIN
OVARY / TESTIS

Respiratory system

The respiratory system includes the mouth, nose, pharynx, larynx, trachea, two bronchi and two lungs (including the bronchioles, alveoli and coverings of the lungs, i.e. the pleura). Also involved in the respiratory process are the muscles of respiration (the intercostal muscles and the diaphragm). The main function of the respiratory system is to take oxygen into the body which is needed for energy-producing reactions and to excrete carbon dioxide, the waste product of these reactions. The exchange of gases between the lungs and the blood is called external respiration, and the exchange of gases between the cells of the body and the blood is called internal respiration.

Asthma

The asthmatic experiences bouts of breathlessness, tightness in the chest and throat, and wheezy breathing. During an asthmatic attack the muscles of the bronchi go into spasm and constrict the airways, and there is also increased mucus production which blocks the airways further. Asthma may be due to an allergy such as to dust, pollen feathers or animals, or may occur in later life in those with a history of respiratory problems. Stress can also be another cause of an asthma attack.

DR: lungs, bronchi

AR: adrenals (for inflammation, stress, allergy), heart (for circulation), solar plexus (for relaxation), sinuses, face (may be affected)

Bronchitis

In the condition of bronchitis, there is inflammation of the bronchi, the tubes that lead from the windpipe to the lungs. This may be associated with infection such as with a cold or influenza, or a chronic condition may result from persistent exposure to irritants such as cigarette smoke, car fumes and other atmospheric pollutants.

DR: lungs, bronchi

AR: thoracic lymphatics (for infection), adrenals (for inflammation), sinus, face (may be affected)

Emphysema

In emphysema there is a wearing out of the elastic tissue of the lungs so that there is a loss of the lungs to spring back into shape after being stretched in inspiration. This results in the lungs remaining partly inflated and the chest stays in a partly expanded position. Symptoms may include shortness of breath, coughing, difficulty in breathing out and, as the condition worsens, a barrel-shaped chest, blue lips and face.

DR: lungs

AR: bronchi (area nearby), thoracic lymphatics (for infection), heart (for circulation), adrenals (for inflammation)

Pleurisy

With pleurisy, there is inflammation of the pleura caused by infection. There are symptoms of pain in the sides of the chest and in the shoulder which are worse when coughing.

DR: lungs

AR: bronchi (area nearby), thoracic lymphatics (for infection), heart (for circulation), adrenals (for inflammation)

Pneumonia

In pneumonia there is inflammation of the lung tissue due to infection, and fluid from the irritated tissues gets into the small air sacs and reduces the amount of usable lung space. There may be symptoms of fever, chest pain and cough.

DR: lungs

AR: bronchi (area nearby), thoracic lymphatics (for infection), adrenals (for inflammation)

HEAD / BRAIN / SINUSES

EUSTACHIAN TUBE
EYE
LUNG
LYMPH DRAINAGE
SIDE OF HEAD / BRAIN
TOP OF HEAD / BRAIN
PITUITARY
ADRENAL
KIDNEY
PARATHYROIDS
NECK
THYROID
STOMACH / PANCREAS
GALL BLADDER
URETER TUBE
BLADDER
SCIATIC

EARS
SHOULDER
SPLEEN   LIVER
TRANSVERSE COLON
WAIST LEVEL
DESCENDING   ASCENDING
COLON   COLON
SMALL INTESTINE
ILEO-CAECAL VALUE
SIGMOID COLON

RIGHT

HEAD / BRAIN / SINUSES

EUSTACHIAN TUBE
EYE
HEART
SOLAR PLEXUS
LYMPH DRAINAGE
TOP OF HEAD / BRAIN
PITUITARY
SIDE OF
HEAD / BRAIN
PARATHYROIDS
NECK
THYROID
STOMACH / PANCREAS
ADRENAL
KIDNEY
URETER TUBE
BLADDER
RECTUM
SCIATIC

LEFT

The respiratory system (PALMS OF THE HANDS)

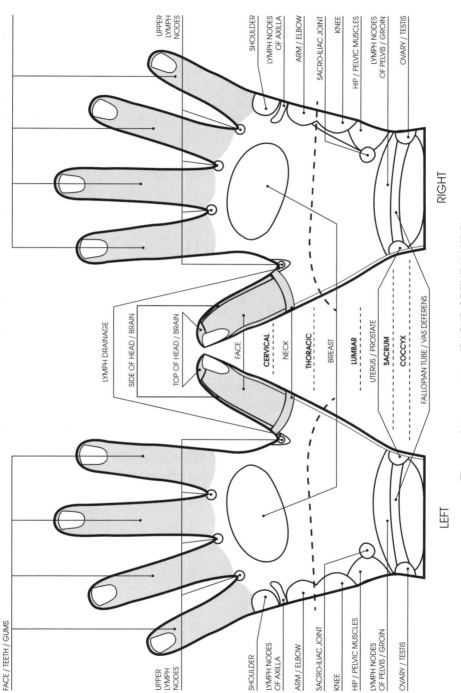

The respiratory system (BACKS OF THE HANDS)

RIGHT

LEFT

FACE / TEETH / GUMS

UPPER LYMPH NODES

SHOULDER

LYMPH NODES OF AXILLA

ARM / ELBOW

SACRO-ILIAC JOINT

KNEE

HIP / PELVIC MUSCLES

LYMPH NODES OF PELVIS / GROIN

OVARY / TESTIS

LYMPH DRAINAGE

SIDE OF HEAD / BRAIN

TOP OF HEAD / BRAIN

FACE

CERVICAL

NECK

THORACIC

BREAST

LUMBAR

UTERUS / PROSTATE

SACRUM

COCCYX

FALLOPIAN TUBE / VAS DEFERENS

UPPER LYMPH NODES

SHOULDER

LYMPH NODES OF AXILLA

ARM / ELBOW

SACRO-ILIAC JOINT

KNEE

HIP / PELVIC MUSCLES

LYMPH NODES OF PELVIS / GROIN

OVARY / TESTIS

Rhinitis and hay fever

With rhinitis there is inflammation of the membranes of the nose due to an allergy to substances such as dust, animal hairs or flowers, and with hay fever the allergy is to grass pollens. The symptoms that present include a streaming nose (or sometimes a blocked nose), sneezing and watering of the eyes. These reactions are due to an oversensitivity of the mucus membranes to substances, and the treatment can help reduce this oversensitivity. Where the allergy is a seasonal one, such as with hay fever, it is best to treat the person before the time of year when they are affected – first to try to reduce the chance of the reaction occurring, and second to prevent making the person much worse when they are already in a bad state.

DR: sinuses, face (nose), eyes

AR: adrenals (for allergy, inflammation), upper lymphatics (for infection)

Sinusitis and catarrh

Many people suffer from congestion in the nose and sinuses probably due to factors such as air pollution, working in air-conditioned offices, double-glazing in houses so that windows are rarely opened and a general lack of fresh air. With sinusitis there may also be pain in the face and around the eyes where the sinuses are positioned. Following treatment it is quite common for the nose and the sinuses to clear and for cold-like symptoms to develop as the excess mucus is cleared. This reaction occurs very readily, and it is important not to overwork the sinus areas when first treating a patient.

DR: sinuses, face (nose)

AR: Eustachian tubes, eyes, adrenals (for inflammation), ileo-caecal valve, large intestine (for elimination), upper lymphatics (for infection)

Sore throat

A sore throat (tonsillitis, laryngitis, pharyngitis, tracheitis) may develop on its own or accompany a cold. It is due to infection. The tonsils are found in the throat in the region called the pharynx and are made up of lymph tissue. They enlarge when infection occurs, and if there are repeated infections they can remain enlarged and become ulcerated. In the condition of tonsillitis, the tonsils become inflamed, and this is more common in children when the tonsils are more active. Laryngitis involves inflammation of the larynx (or voice box), and when this occurs the voice is affected and may even be lost temporarily.

DR: face, throat

AR: upper lymphatics (for infection), sinuses, adrenals (for inflammation)

Cardiovascular system

The cardiovascular system includes the heart and blood vessels (arteries, capillaries and veins). The heart is responsible for pumping blood around the body and blood is the major transport system for oxygen, carbon dioxide, nutrients, hormones, heat, protective substances (e.g. antibodies) and blood-clotting factors.

Angina

With angina, a person experiences short, sharp pains in the chest region where the heart is situated, usually following some exertion. This occurs due to decreased blood supply and therefore a lack of oxygen to the heart muscle.

DR: heart

AR: solar plexus (for relaxation), adrenals (for increased blood flow, stress), lungs (for breathing)

The cardiovascular system (PALMS OF THE HANDS)

LEFT

RIGHT

HEAD / BRAIN / SINUSES

HEAD / BRAIN / SINUSES

EUSTACHIAN TUBE
EYE
HEART
SOLAR PLEXUS
LYMPH DRAINAGE
TOP OF HEAD / BRAIN
PITUITARY
SIDE OF HEAD / BRAIN
PARATHYROIDS
NECK
THYROID
STOMACH / PANCREAS
ADRENAL
KIDNEY
URETER TUBE
BLADDER
RECTUM
SCIATIC

EARS
SHOULDER
SPLEEN   LIVER
TRANSVERSE COLON
WAIST LEVEL
DESCENDING COLON   ASCENDING COLON
SMALL INTESTINE
ILEO-CAECAL VALVE
SIGMOID COLON

EUSTACHIAN TUBE
EYE
LUNG
LYMPH DRAINAGE
SIDE OF HEAD / BRAIN
TOP OF HEAD / BRAIN
PITUITARY
ADRENAL
KIDNEY
PARATHYROIDS
NECK
THYROID
STOMACH / PANCREAS
GALL BLADDER
URETER TUBE
BLADDER
SCIATIC

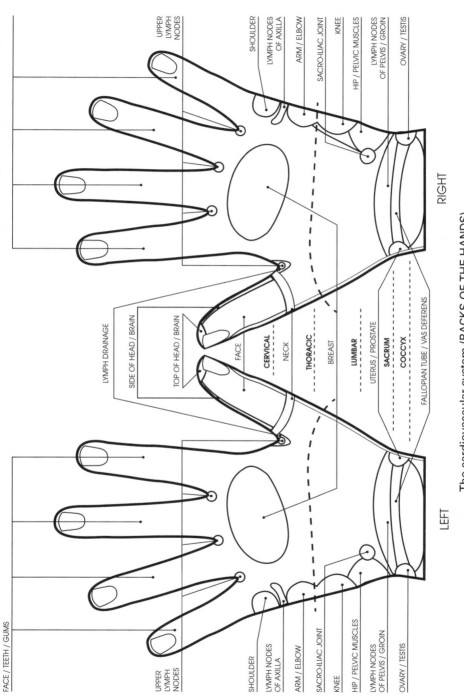

FACE / TEETH / GUMS

SHOULDER
LYMPH NODES OF AXILLA
ARM / ELBOW
SACRO-ILIAC JOINT
KNEE
HIP / PELVIC MUSCLES
LYMPH NODES OF PELVIS / GROIN
OVARY / TESTIS

UPPER LYMPH NODES

LYMPH DRAINAGE
SIDE OF HEAD / BRAIN
TOP OF HEAD / BRAIN
FACE
CERVICAL
NECK
THORACIC
BREAST
LUMBAR
UTERUS / PROSTATE
SACRUM
COCCYX
FALLOPIAN TUBE / VAS DEFERENS

UPPER LYMPH NODES

SHOULDER
LYMPH NODES OF AXILLA
ARM / ELBOW
SACRO-ILIAC JOINT
KNEE
HIP / PELVIC MUSCLES
LYMPH NODES OF PELVIS / GROIN
OVARY / TESTIS

RIGHT

LEFT

The cardiovascular system (BACKS OF THE HANDS)

Anaemia

With anaemia there is a reduced level of red blood cells and thus decreased haemoglobin such that the transport of oxygen to the cells is reduced. Symptoms may include tiredness, lack of energy, shortness of breath and a pale complexion. The most common cause is a deficiency of iron, though it may also be linked to a lack of vitamin B12 or folate in the body.

DR: heart

AR: spleen (for breakdown of red blood cells), stomach (for vitamin B12 absorption), lungs (for oxygen availability)

Arteriosclerosis

With arteriosclerosis the blood vessels that carry oxygen and nutrients become thick and stiff, which can restrict blood flow to organs and tissues. A specific type of arteriosclerosis is atherosclerosis whereby fats, cholesterol and other substance build up on the artery walls forming plaque (atheroma), which reduces blood flow in the area. It can also cause the arteries to narrow and harden, and the plaque might rupture to cause a blood clot. This would result in a stroke if occurring in the brain or a heart attack if occurring in the heart.

DR: heart

AR: areas affected (e.g. knee for lower leg), adrenals (for increased blood flow, stress)

Chilblains

Poor circulation can lead to chilblains whereby red, oval swellings appear on the fingers or toes, which are intensely itchy. These swellings appear when the areas get cold, especially if it is also damp. Problems with nerve supply from the spine may be involved with the upper spine if the fingers are affected and the lower spine if the toes are affected. Poor elimination through the digestive tract may be causing congestion in the body, affecting circulation.

DR: arm (for hand), knee (for foot)

AR: heart (for circulation), adrenals (for increased blood flow), spine (for nerve supply), small intestine, large intestine, liver (for elimination), zone-related areas (e.g. toes for fingers)

Hypertension

One of the common causes of hypertension (high blood pressure) is stress, though other factors may include obesity, heart or kidney disease and dietary factors such as excess alcohol and smoking. Symptoms that may be experienced include headaches, dizziness, ringing in the ears, breathlessness, chest pain and cough, and the eyesight may be affected. In some cases, a person may have high blood pressure without being aware of any symptoms. Where high blood pressure is present there is added strain on the heart, blood vessels and kidneys.

DR: heart

AR: adrenals (for stress and hormonal effect on blood pressure), kidneys, pituitary (influence blood pressure), head/brain (if there are headaches), ears (if there is tinnitus), eyes (if there are eye problems), solar plexus (for relaxation)

Hypotension

Some people normally have hypotension (low blood pressure), but it can also occur as a complication of another disorder (e.g. if a person is in shock, has Addison's disease, has a haemorrhage). The condition leads to an inadequate blood supply to the brain, which could lead to dizziness, fainting or unconsciousness.

DR: heart

AR: adrenals (for stress, influence blood pressure and if affected, e.g. Addison's disease), head/brain (if affected), pituitary, kidneys (influence blood pressure)

Palpitations

Palpitations are when the heart is beating more forcefully and faster to the extent that the person becomes aware of their heart beating. Palpitations may be associated with anxiety or stress or be associated with an overactive thyroid gland.

DR: heart

AR: solar plexus (for relaxation), adrenals (for stress), thyroid (for hormonal balance)

Raynaud's disease

In Raynaud's disease the arteries in the hands (or feet) go into spasm and tighten when cold, with the fingers going pale and dead, and then red and swollen. As the fingers warm there may be a burning and tingling sensation.

DR: arm (for hand)

AR: heart (for circulation), adrenals (for increased blood flow), spine (for nerve supply), small intestine, large intestine, liver (for elimination), zone-related areas (e.g. toes for fingers)

Varicose veins

Varicose veins commonly occur in the legs whereby the veins become swollen and twisted. They may also be painful. They occur more as people get older but are more likely to occur in those who are overweight or who stand for long periods. Although it is unlikely that reflexology treatment will get rid of existing varicose veins, it may be able to ease the discomfort felt and also improve the circulation to help prevent the formation of additional varicose veins. Problems with the nerve supply from the lower spine may be involved or poor elimination through the digestive tract may be causing congestion in the body, affecting circulation. A complication of varicose veins could be the formation of blood clots resulting in thrombophlebitis or deep vein thrombosis. Venous leg ulcers are another potential problem.

DR: parts affected (e.g. knee for lower leg)

AR: heart (for circulation), adrenals (for inflammation), spine (for nerve supply), small intestine, large intestine, liver (for elimination)

Lymphatic system

The lymphatic system includes the lymph vessels distributed throughout the body, lymph nodes, spleen, thymus, tonsils and adenoids, and appendix. The main functions of the lymphatic system are to help fight infection and to drain excess fluid from the tissues.

Acquired immune deficiency syndrome

Acquired immune deficiency syndrome (AIDS) results from the presence of the human immunodeficiency virus (HIV) in the body. This attacks a weakened immune system and gives rise to AIDS, which may start with flu-like symptoms but then progresses with the development of infections in other parts of the body such as pneumonia, diarrhoea and weight loss due to infection in the digestive tract, as well as skin eruptions.

DR: lymphatics, spleen

AR: lungs, large intestine (if affected), adrenals (for inflammation, stress), solar plexus (for relaxation)

Allergies

Many people suffer from allergies. When allergies develop in the body there is an oversensitivity of a part of the body to certain substances. This may involve areas such as the digestive tract, in the form of food allergies, the skin, causing eczema, or the lungs, causing asthma, or affecting the head to cause migraines. Reflexology treatment helps to reduce the oversensitivity in the body and thus helps to reduce the allergic response.

DR: adrenals, spleen, lymphatics

AR: stomach, large intestine (for food allergy), lungs (for respiratory allergy such as asthma, hay fever), head/brain (for headache, migraine)

The lymphatic system (PALMS OF THE HANDS)

HEAD / BRAIN / SINUSES

EUSTACHIAN TUBE
EYE
LUNG
LYMPH DRAINAGE
SIDE OF HEAD / BRAIN
TOP OF HEAD / BRAIN
PITUITARY
ADRENAL
KIDNEY
PARATHYROIDS
NECK
THYROID
STOMACH / PANCREAS
GALL BLADDER
URETER TUBE
BLADDER
SCIATIC

RIGHT

EARS
SHOULDER
SPLEEN   LIVER
TRANSVERSE COLON
WAIST LEVEL
DESCENDING   ASCENDING
COLON   COLON
SMALL INTESTINE
ILEO-CAECAL VALUE
SIGMOID COLON

LEFT

HEAD / BRAIN / SINUSES

EUSTACHIAN TUBE
EYE
HEART
SOLAR PLEXUS
LYMPH DRAINAGE
TOP OF HEAD / BRAIN
PITUITARY
SIDE OF HEAD / BRAIN
PARATHYROIDS
NECK
THYROID
STOMACH / PANCREAS
ADRENAL
KIDNEY
URETER TUBE
BLADDER
RECTUM
SCIATIC

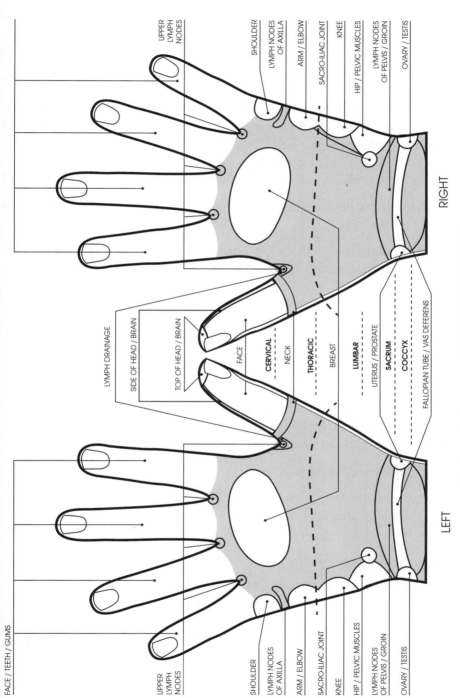

FACE / TEETH / GUMS

UPPER
LYMPH
NODES

SHOULDER

LYMPH NODES
OF AXILLA

ARM / ELBOW

SACRO-ILIAC JOINT

KNEE

HIP / PELVIC MUSCLES

LYMPH NODES
OF PELVIS / GROIN

OVARY / TESTIS

LYMPH DRAINAGE

SIDE OF HEAD / BRAIN

TOP OF HEAD / BRAIN

FACE

CERVICAL

NECK

THORACIC

BREAST

LUMBAR

UTERUS / PROSTATE

SACRUM

COCCYX

FALLOPIAN TUBE / VAS DEFERENS

UPPER
LYMPH
NODES

SHOULDER

LYMPH NODES
OF AXILLA

ARM / ELBOW

SACRO-ILIAC JOINT

KNEE

HIP / PELVIC MUSCLES

LYMPH NODES
OF PELVIS / GROIN

OVARY / TESTIS

RIGHT

LEFT

The lymphatic system (BACKS OF THE HANDS)

Cancer

Cancer cells develop in the body when the body's own defence system is unable to destroy them, and these cells can settle in many different areas such as the lungs, cervix, breast, stomach and large intestine (colon). Reflexology can be used in conjunction with other natural therapies and orthodox treatments to try to help strengthen the body's immune system. Where orthodox treatment is being received, treatment may help the body cope with some of the side effects experienced. Treatment can also be given to those seriously ill with cancer to help with relaxation, pain relief and general well-being.

DR: parts affected (e.g. lungs, uterus, breasts, stomach, large intestine)

AR: lymphatics, spleen (to strengthen immune system) solar plexus (relaxation), adrenals (for inflammation, stress)

Infections

Infections of different parts of the body occur when the body's own defence system is not strong enough to overcome the infection. General conditions, such as influenza, may result, or more specific infections such as ear infections or bladder infections. Reflexology treatment may help to clear an infection but more importantly may help to strengthen the body's defence system to prevent infections from occurring in the future.

DR: parts affected (e.g. lungs, sinuses, ears, bladder)

AR: lymphatics, spleen (for infection), adrenals (for inflammation)

Lymphoedema

With lymphoedema there is swelling in the body's tissues which most commonly involves the arms or legs. Because of the swelling, the affected area may feel heavy and difficult to move. It is caused by a problem with the lymphatic system, which is either genetic or from damage to the system such as from infection, injury or cancer treatment.

DR: arm, knee, hip (for leg)

AR: lymphatics, spleen (to strengthen system), kidneys (for elimination), adrenals (for inflammation)

Systemic lupus erythematosus

Systemic lupus erythematosus (commonly referred to as lupus) can affect many parts of the body such as the skin, joints and internal organs. Symptoms vary, and with lupus the most common symptoms are extreme tiredness, skin rashes (especially on the face, wrists and hands), joint pain and swelling. It is thought to be an autoimmune disorder that may be due to genetic and environmental factors.

DR: parts affected (face, knee, hip)

AR: lymphatics, spleen (to strengthen immune system), adrenals (for inflammation, allergies, stress), solar plexus (relaxation)

Myalgic Encephalomyelitis (M.E.)

With the condition of M.E., chronic fatigue syndrome or post-viral syndrome, the person develops extreme fatigue and muscle weakness following an infection and this can last for months or years after the infection has cleared. There may also be disturbances of the digestive system. Sometimes when a course of treatment is commenced, a person with M.E. can feel more tired after treatment, but this effect will soon pass.

DR: lymphatics, spleen

AR: adrenals (for inflammation, stress, allergy), head/brain (for depression), stomach, small intestine, large intestine (for digestive problems)

Thrush

Thrush (or candidiasis) is a yeast infection caused by a fungus, *Candida albicans*. It can affect both women and men, with vaginal thrush in women being most common, but it may also affect the head of the penis in men or, with oral thrush, the mouth is affected. The area affected is sore and red with a discharge. Reflexology treatment may help to prevent recurring thrush by strengthening the immune system.

DR: parts affected (vagina, throat, penis)

AR: lymphatics, spleen (to fight infection), adrenals (for inflammation)

The conditions mentioned above are some of the more common conditions that might present for reflexology treatment. There are very few conditions where reflexology treatment would be a complete contraindication, though with quite a number of conditions extra care would be required by the practitioner depending on the individual situation. These conditions are discussed in Chapter 7.

Chapter 7

When to Use Reflexology and When Not to Use It

Chapter 6 looks at a large number of conditions which the reflexology practitioner might come across and about which he or she should therefore have an understanding. There are other conditions that have not been described but which might be helped, and the necessary approach to treatment may well be similar to some of those described. It should always be remembered that reflexology will not replace orthodox medicine for more serious conditions but can often be used as a safe complementary therapy alongside orthodox medicine. In addition, it is not possible to diagnose disorders with reflexology – only reflex areas out of balance – and a client should always be encouraged to see a medical practitioner for a medical diagnosis.

Contraindications to reflexology treatment

There are a few conditions for which reflexology treatment would not be appropriate including the following:

- acute infectious diseases – when there would also be a risk of the practitioner catching the infection

- fevers, very high temperatures – the body should be allowed to try to fight the infection initially or for medication to be taken if necessary

- acute inflammation of the venous system such as with deep vein thrombosis or thrombophlebitis or the presence of an aneurysm – there is a risk of moving a blood clot to an area where there might be a more serious consequence (though there is no evidence to suggest that reflexology treatment might move a blood clot) or where an aneurysm might rupture

- severe osteoporosis whereby the bones of the hand are affected – there would be a risk of damaging a brittle bone if applying massage

- directly after replacement surgery, such as for a new hip or new heart valve – there is always a risk of rejection of a new part by the body and it is best to wait until it has been established that the new part has been accepted so as not to interfere with this process

- directly before major surgery – there is always a risk of a healing reaction to a first reflexology treatment, so it would not be appropriate for this to be given immediately prior to surgery

- immediately before medical tests – giving reflexology treatment might distort the test results

- after inoculations – it is best not to give treatment for a period of 48 hours following inoculations to allow the inoculation to be effective so as not to increase any adverse reaction to the inoculation

- those in a severely disturbed mental state or suffering from psychosis and those under the influence of drugs and/or alcohol – there might be a risk to the practitioner.

Extra care when giving treatment

There are several instances when the practitioner would need to be extra cautious, especially when first treating a client as some clients can show a strong reaction to treatment. These situations might include the following:

- a client who is taking medication when, as a result of reflexology treatment, medication may need to be adjusted (e.g. for diabetes, thyroid problems, high blood pressure)

- a client who is taking medication (e.g. pain killers, tranquillisers, antidepressants) that may mask the sensitivity of the reflexes

- a client with a heart condition – so as not to overstimulate the heart

- a client who has epilepsy – reflexology treatment might cause an epileptic fit, though this is uncommon

- a client who has a prostheses – there is always a slight risk that an artificial part present in the body (e.g. contact lenses, replacement joints, replacement heart valves, pacemaker, intrauterine contraceptive device) may be rejected and that reflexology treatment might encourage this

- a client who is receiving other therapies, particularly if they have just started receiving this therapy – there is the possibility of a healing reaction from many complementary therapies and this might be exaggerated if more than one type of treatment was received, and also the client will not know which treatment is beneficial if they show improvement.

Reflexology treatment for all age groups

Reflexology treatment is appropriate for all age groups, from the very young to the very old, and for both males and females.

Children

Children of all ages may benefit from reflexology treatment. Hand reflexology may be particularly useful with youngsters since it takes less time than foot reflexology and may be a better option if a child finds that one hour of foot reflexology is too long to sit still (also if they think their feet might be ticklish). In babies, it may be helpful for such conditions as colic, teething, eczema and sleep problems. In children, treatment can be helpful for any of the conditions previously described, and the most common conditions seen include asthma, eczema, digestive problems and frequent colds and coughs. It may be necessary when treating a very young child to use slightly lighter pressure than usual when applying the massage, but all the reflex areas can be precisely worked. At time of puberty, it should be remembered that the reflex areas to the hormonal system may be particularly sensitive as the body adjusts to the changes taking place with this system, so it is important not to overwork these areas.

Elderly adults

Hand reflexology is a very appropriate treatment for the elderly and is often greatly enjoyed by elderly people. An elderly client may consider regular reflexology treatment as a means of maintaining a good level of health, but for those less well, specific conditions may be eased even if it is not possible to clear them totally. For those in a care home or a nursing home, reflexology treatment is often made available.

One of the greatest benefits of treatment to the elderly is the one-to-one contact with the practitioner and the presence of touch by massage to the hands, which is comforting to an elderly person. These are added benefits to those of treatment for specific conditions. Hand reflexology treatment can often be more appropriate than foot reflexology treatment for an older person, who might find the process of removing footwear difficult or slow. Also, it might be easier for them to concentrate on the shorter treatment of hand reflexology. The position for treatment may also be more appropriate with the client being able to sit in a comfortable chair rather than in a reclining position or even sitting or lying on a bed.

When working with elderly or frail clients it may be necessary to use lighter pressure and to be aware that the skin may be finer, with possible skin imperfections. Also, as the person is older, there is a greater possibility of deterioration in many of the body systems and therefore there may be a number of sensitive reflex areas. If there is arthritis in the hands, it might be that working directly on the hands causes more pain and therefore would not be appropriate. If the client is diabetic, there may be reduced sensitivity in the hands with finer skin that bruises more easily, and there may also be reduced healing capacity. If there is heart disease, the treatment may help circulation generally and could still be given, even if the person has had heart surgery. In any case, treatment is usually possible and can have many benefits. Hand reflexology for the elderly is possibly one of the most useful and widely used areas for this particular type of treatment.

Adults in general

Although a wide range of conditions in adults have already been discussed, some particular conditions (which often also apply to adolescents) are considered below.

PREGNANCY

Reflexology can be a useful treatment to a pregnant woman, and maternity reflexology has become a popular area of reflexology with courses being run to provide additional information to practitioners, particularly with regard to a more detailed look at the physiology of pregnancy and possible conditions that can develop during this time. However, a well-trained practitioner should have the necessary skills to treat a woman who is pregnant.

Treatment might be a contraindication in the early stages of pregnancy if the client had never had reflexology before and when it is the first pregnancy or when there has been a previous miscarriage. However, for most women, reflexology can be safely given throughout pregnancy.

Some women consider a short course of treatment leading up to the time they are due to give birth to encourage the baby to arrive on time and for the birth to be straightforward. It is also possible for a midwife to use reflexology points to help with labour. Following childbirth a woman may experience post-natal symptoms as the body and hormonal levels readjust. There may be symptoms such as tiredness, depression, urinary tract infection, problems with breastfeeding and discomfort in the breasts. These symptoms may well be helped by giving extra attention to the appropriate reflex areas such as the ovaries, uterus, pituitary (for readjustment of the reproductive system and hormones), head/brain (for depression), bladder, ureter tubes, kidneys, lymphatics (for urinary infections) and breasts (for breast problems).

CANCER

There are many examples of reflexology treatment being used to treat cancer patients and there are now an increasing number of hospitals offering complementary therapies to cancer patients. Complementary therapies including reflexology are also treatments made available by a hospice. It is important for the practitioner to be aware of the medical treatment being received and likely reactions that this might produce, and to be particularly careful to prevent strong healing reactions.

Reflexology treatment can be given to those receiving orthodox treatment (though it is best to receive consent for this from the client's medical practitioner), and the best time to treat will depend on how orthodox treatment is being administered. Some clients like reflexology treatment before their orthodox treatment as it helps them to be more relaxed and to sleep better prior to their treatment.

In addition to a full treatment, extra attention may be given to the reflex areas to the affected parts (e.g. breast, head, colon) and to the lymphatics and spleen (for immune system), liver, kidneys, large intestine (for elimination), solar plexus (for relaxation) and adrenals (for stress).

For those recovering from cancer, reflexology may help this process, and regular treatment may keep the body in balance and prevent a reoccurrence of their cancer. For those who may be terminally ill, treatment may also be given to help general well-being, relaxation, aid sleep and reduce stress.

ADDICTIONS

Reflexology can sometimes be of help to those trying to overcome addictions. For those trying to give up smoking, reflexology may be helpful, together with other positive steps, to aid relaxation and help reduce cravings. As a result of reflexology treatment, a person often feels better in themselves which may possibly reduce the desire to smoke. Working on the reflex areas to the head/brain areas may help, together with the solar plexus (for relaxation), adrenals (for stress) and the areas to the respiratory system (to clear the effects of smoking on this system).

For those trying to come off drugs or wanting to reduce medication, such as tranquillisers, in conjunction with appropriate medical care, reflexology may help with relaxation, well-being and encourage the body to clear toxins from the body systems. The reflex area to the liver may be particularly sensitive in these cases, so it should not be overworked.

EATING DISORDERS

There is a growing increase in the number of people with obesity, and being obese can lead to a greater risk of diabetes, heart disease and some types of cancer. The condition can also lead to low self-esteem and depression. The major cause of obesity is overeating, though there can be physical causes. Whilst reflexology treatment will not by itself cause weight loss, treatment may help a person who is trying to lose weight by reducing their food intake, by helping with relaxation and stress, and by improving general well-being, which might in turn lead to a reduced desire to overeat.

The eating disorders anorexia nervosa and bulimia do require specialist help, but reflexology may complement this by helping with relaxation, stress and general well-being. It also helps balance the functioning of the digestive system which may be of particular benefit when a person is overcoming these conditions.

Pain management

Pain is a reaction in the body that something is wrong. It may be acute or chronic. Acute pain generally comes on suddenly as a result of injury to a part such as a joint injury, inflammation of an area such as toothache or disease of a part such as a chest infection. Although stressful at the time, once treatment of the cause has been successful, the pain disappears. Chronic pain persists over a period of time, causing much distress to the person, and results from an injury or disease that cannot be completely treated successfully, and which therefore is persistently present. Reflexology may help with easing pain in these conditions with the effectiveness of treatment varying in length from a few hours following treatment to a few days or weeks. Important reflex areas to treat for pain include the area to the part affected, plus reflex areas to the head/brain and spine. The brain has systems to help reduce pain and will send messages via the spinal cord and then along nerves to the part affected to help reduce pain.

Self-treatment

Hand reflexology can be easily applied to oneself, and in many ways self-treatment to the hands is more easily administered than self-treatment to the feet. A practitioner may also recommend that a client do some work on their own hands in between treatment sessions, though this would not be advised if a serious condition were present such as a heart problem, diabetes or thyroid imbalance, whereby there might be the risk of the client overworking areas. Often a client will ask if they can treat themselves in between treatment, and showing them a few areas that can be easily located involves the client in the healing process.

Self-treatment may also be beneficial to ease occasional symptoms such as a stiff neck (neck reflex), lower back pain (spine reflex), sciatica (sciatic reflex), blocked and painful ears during takeoff or landing when flying (ear and Eustachian tube reflexes) when the individual reflex areas could be worked. For those without knowledge of the positions of the reflex areas, working up and down the zones on both the palm side and back of the hand may bring some benefit as all of the body will be treated, though not as precisely as with hand reflexology treatment.

Hand reflexology can also be used by practitioners when giving a demonstration of treatment, and depending on the time available, either a full treatment could be given or a shorter version. A shorter version could include work on areas which are commonly affected or are useful in many cases and are easy to locate. This might include working on the reflex areas of the thumbs (for the pituitary, neck and head), spine, fingers (for the head and sinuses), solar plexus (for relaxation), adrenals (for inflammation, stress or allergy), large intestine and kidneys (for elimination), and lymphatics (for the immune system). It would be sensible to work these areas on both hands for balance.

Staying healthy

It is not necessary to be unwell to receive reflexology treatment. Regular treatment can help maintain good health and prevent imbalances from occurring, and the relaxation effect of reflexology treatment will be of benefit to everyone. With the hands so accessible and treatment not taking very long, hand reflexology treatment can be given so easily – perhaps when on the train or the bus, whilst a passenger in a car or whilst watching television. By treating the whole body through the hands on a regular basis, not only will body systems be encouraged to work efficiently, this may also help contribute to such things as healthy hair and nails (buffing the fingertips may stimulate hair growth) and even produce an anti-ageing effect – a much sought-after panacea!

Chapter 8

Conditions Affecting the Hands

As the hands are to be worked on with hand reflexology, it would be expected for the practitioner to be aware of some of the common conditions that can affect the hands themselves, and which might therefore be seen. Some of these conditions are mentioned in Chapter 6 as conditions that might be helped by reflexology, but some of the conditions are ones for which reflexology would not be the most appropriate form of treatment. Although reflexology is not a diagnostic treatment, it would, however, be useful to know about some of the hand conditions that might be seen.

Arthritis

Arthritis in the hands is quite common with pain and inflammation of a joint or joints. The most common sites affected are:

- the base of the thumb – a deep aching pain may be felt which is often worse from activities that involve a pinching action such as opening jars, turning door knobs or keys, and writing

- the metacarpophalangeal joints – these are the large joints at the base of the fingers which act as hinge joints and are important for both power grip and pinch activities, and these activities are reduced when arthritis is present

- osteoarthritis – in this condition, the cushioning cartilage covering the bone surface at joints begins to wear out and the joint becomes swollen and painful

- rheumatoid arthritis – in this condition there is an effect on cells lining and lubricating the joints, which become swollen and painful.

Carpal tunnel syndrome

In carpal tunnel syndrome there is an increased pressure on the median nerve at the wrist (pinched nerve), which can result in weakness, pain and tingling in the hand, and this may radiate to the forearm and shoulder.

Cubital tunnel syndrome

In cubital tunnel syndrome there is an increased pressure on the ulnar nerve at the elbow.

Dupuytren's disease

In Dupuytren's disease there is an abnormal thickening of the fascia in the palm of the hand which often starts with firm lumps or nodules in the palm. The nodules can then extend and form cords of tissue which contract and then pull on the fingers, to which they are connected, causing the fingers to bend towards the palm.

Ganglion cysts

A ganglion is a fluid-filled cyst that develops adjacent to a joint or tendon. It may be quite small (the size of a pea) or quite large (the size of a golf ball). Common sites for a ganglion to occur are the wrist (particularly the back of the wrist), hand and fingers.

Gout

Gout is a form of arthritis that occurs when there is a build-up of uric acid in the blood due to overproduction or defective excretion by the kidneys, with sodium urate crystals being deposited in the joints and tendons. In pseudo-gout, crystals of calcium pyrophosphate are deposited. The affected joint is painful, shiny, swollen and red. The thumb may be affected and sometimes the wrist.

Mallet finger

Mallet finger involves deformity of a finger caused by damage to the extensor tendon to the finger. The end of the finger bends in the direction of the palm and the finger cannot be straightened at the end since the tendon is stretched or torn. The finger is often painful and swollen. It is often caused by a minor injury such as catching the finger on an item, or can be a common sports injury when the end of the finger is struck by a ball or other object.

Trigger finger

Trigger finger, also known as stenosing tenosynovitis, involves the tendons in hand that bend the fingers. One or more fingers may be affected and the finger or thumb is bent towards the palm, and the tendon gets stuck causing the finger to click or lock. The symptoms may include pain, stiffness, clicking and the formation of a small nodule in the palm at the base of the affected finger.

Fractures

A fracture is where there is a break in the continuity of a bone. It is possible to fracture the bones in the hand and this is common following a fall when the hand is often used to try to break the fall, or due to sports injury. Common sites in the hand for a fracture are the fingers, scaphoid bone and wrist. There is an increased risk of fractures in women after menopause whereby there can be rapid bone loss leading to osteoporosis.

Skin conditions

Conditions such as eczema, psoriasis and dermatitis are all described in Chapter 6, and these conditions can affect the hands. Very often a skin problem on the hands can be linked to an allergy to something that the hands are coming into contact with such as soap, hand cream, washing powder or detergent. The condition of vitiligo in which there is a patchy loss of pigmentation of the skin, possibly caused by an autoimmune condition, can also affect the hands. Warts (*verrucae*) can also be present on the hands.

Circulatory problems

If there are circulatory problems, the hands are often the parts affected, being a distant part from the heart, which is pumping blood around the body. Cold hands may become a particular problem in the winter months, and other problems may also develop such as chilblains and Raynaud's disease (both described in Chapter 6).

Chapter 9

Different Approaches to Hand Reflexology

Vertical Reflex Therapy

Vertical Reflex Therapy (VRT) for the hands and feet was discovered and developed by reflexologist Lynne Booth in the early 1990s. This newer reflexology technique is a radical change from the traditional image of a reflexologist working on the plantar surface of the feet or palm of the hands as it is the dorsal reflexes on the weight-bearing hands and feet that are stimulated systematically for up to five minutes, usually at the start and finish of a classical reflexology session. However, both approaches are therapeutic and compatible.

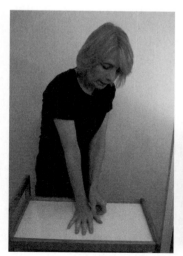
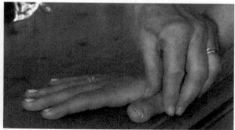

Vertical Reflex Therapy

Analysis: VRT and the possible increase in therapeutic reaction

VRT research indicates that *all* reflexes can be accessed through the dorsum of the hands or feet and that the body is more responsive to some reflexology techniques when briefly treated in a standing or weight-bearing hand position. Anatomically, the nerves in the hands and feet remain desensitised when passive or reclining, and those same nerves become sensitised when the feet are standing or the hands are pressed down on a flat surface. When a reflexologist stimulates the feet, an energetic response appears to be carried through the body to a particular target. It appears obvious that, in the reflexology concept, the response is transmitted in some way by the nerves and, if this is the case, there is a possibility that the *sensitised* weight-bearing reflexes may enhance the response of the stimulated reflex.

VRT may be used as a brief first-aid treatment, as part of a classical reflexology session or as a shortened complete VRT treatment of 20–30 minutes, which is suitable for everyone including children, older people, sport-oriented persons or in the workplace. Brief self-help on the hands for 'homework' between treatments can also be offered to clients.

The role of VRT is seen as complementary to conventional reflexology, although it has been suggested that VRT can often reach deeper reflexes allowing homeostasis to be achieved in a shorter time. In 2002 a small study into *VRT in the workplace* indicated an 80% improvement in some conditions in only four weeks when selected employees were also given a few minutes of VRT 'homework' on specific hand reflexes each day.

Versatility of VRT

One of the reasons VRT has become well integrated into reflexology practice in the UK and internationally is that it is relatively simple for practitioners and their clients to learn, and they have the option of working their own weight-bearing hands between treatments for a few minutes a day. Weight-bearing reflexes tend to be a little more sensitive, but this mild discomfort is compensated by the speed in which relief is sometimes gained from chronic conditions. Mobility and musculoskeletal conditions tend to respond the quickest, and an immediate decrease in pain and increase in mobility has often been experienced.

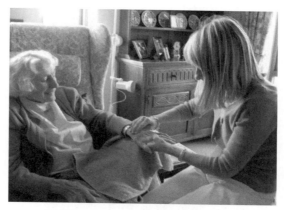

A VRT treatment being administered

All ages and conditions can benefit from VRT, but Lynne Booth was encouraged by the response from chronically ill older clients, with multiple pathologies, at the St Monica Trust, Bristol, and she deduced that if this age group of people could respond so well, then the weight-bearing techniques would be very effective for everyone.

VRT can be applied to the weight-bearing or semi-weight-bearing hands if the client is sitting or even lying (as they can press down on a hard surface such as a small tray or book). To stand for VRT on the feet or press the arm downwards on a flat surface to weight-bear is obviously not so relaxing for the practitioner or client, but it is compensated by the fact that VRT is applied in this position for a maximum of five minutes only, and often two to three minutes is sufficient.

Synergistic reflexology

The first VRT treatments were directed towards musculoskeletal problems, but all conditions can benefit, and subsequently other techniques were developed that include Synergistic Reflexology (SR), where the hand and foot are worked simultaneously to increase the stimulation and efficacy of the reflexes.

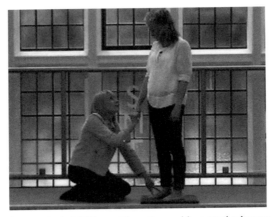

Synergistic VRT working the ankle zonal trigger

Further developments include working three weight-bearing reflexes at once, which incorporates the newly discovered zonal trigger reflexes situated on the wrists and ankles. These reflexes are particularly relevant for longstanding and intransigent problems. Many documented examples illustrating the immediate benefits of VRT have come after the therapist has selected a priority reflex to stimulate on the foot (e.g. a shoulder point) and, at the same time, located a tender reflex on the ankle in the same zone and worked them together with the corresponding reflex on the hand for 30 seconds per foot.

Nail working

Later developments include precise VRT nail working where the toenails and fingernails are worked in conjunction with the dorsal reflexes. It is an effective technique that taps into the inherent pressure on all the reflexes situated under the nails, especially the thumb and big-toe nails. Initially Lynne Booth identified the five Ingham zones on the thumbnails and mapped out sets of reflexes for each system of the body on the dorsum (i.e. on the big-toe nails and thumbnails instead of the traditional tiny zones on the thumb and toe pads).

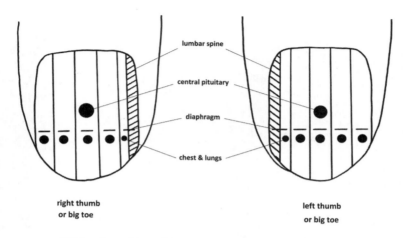

lumbar spine

central pituitary

diaphragm

chest & lungs

right thumb
or big toe

left thumb
or big toe

VRT nail working: focusing on the respiratory system

How often to treat?

Weekly VRT/reflexology treatments produce good results, and a maximum of two sessions per week, in chronic cases, are recommended as the client's body needs time to adjust. Acute cases respond well to daily sessions, and the extremely responsive weight-bearing self-help on the hands and feet can be used several times daily on demand.

Background to the discovery of VRT

Reflexologists are aware that there can be mobility difficulties when working the plantar side of the feet with some disabled clients, and for sheer necessity Lynne Booth began to often work the dorsum of the feet as they rested on the wheelchair supports. Instead of compromising her treatments, she got better results and so mapped out the plantar reflexes on the dorsum as the Ingham Zone theory, which states that the body comprises ten three-dimensional zones, concentrates on the plantar surface. These zones act as conduits for energy that runs from the foot and hand reflexes to specific parts of the body. Zone 1 runs from the thumb or big toe and so on through to zone 5, which runs from the little toe and finger. Booth therefore argued that there is no reason why the reflexes for the body cannot be approached in the same three-dimensional manner from either side of the foot or hands. All reflexes can be accessed through the dorsum of the hand or foot.

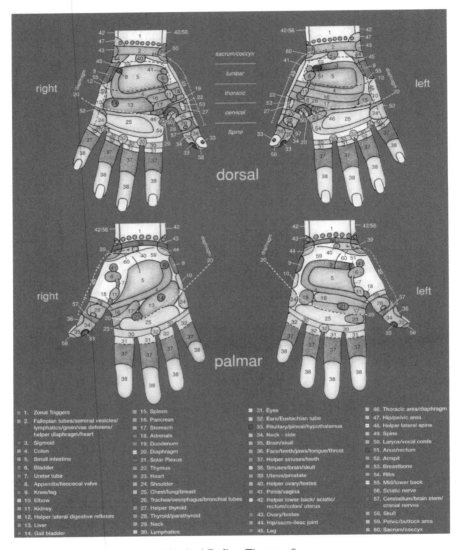

Vertical Reflex Therapy®:
The Booth Method® Hand Chart

1. Zonal Triggers	15. Spleen	31. Eyes	46. Thoracic area/diaphragm
2. Fallopian tubes/seminal vesicles/ lymphatics/groin/vas deferens/ helper diaphragm/heart	16. Pancreas	32. Ears/Eustachian tube	47. Hip/pelvic area
	17. Stomach	33. Pituitary/pineal/hypothalamus	48. Helper lateral spine
	18. Adrenals	34. Neck - side	49. Spine
3. Sigmoid	19. Duodenum	35. Brain/skull	50. Larynx/vocal cords
4. Colon	20. Diaphragm	36. Face/teeth/jaws/tongue/throat	51. Anus/rectum
5. Small intestine	21. Solar Plexus	37. Helper sinuses/teeth	52. Armpit
6. Bladder	22. Thymus	38. Sinuses/brain/skull	53. Breastbone
7. Ureter tube	23. Heart	39. Uterus/prostate	54. Ribs
8. Appendix/ileocecal valve	24. Shoulder	40. Helper ovary/testes	55. Mid/lower back
9. Knee/leg	25. Chest/lung/breast	41. Penis/vagina	56. Sciatic nerve
10. Elbow	26. Trachea/oesophagus/bronchial tubes	42. Helper lower back/ sciatic/ rectum/colon/ uterus	57. Cerebellum/brain stem/ cranial nerves
11. Kidney	27. Helper thyroid		58. Skull
12. Helper lateral digestive reflexes	28. Thyroid/parathyroid	43. Ovary/testes	59. Pelvic/buttock area
13. Liver	29. Neck	44. Hip/sacro-ileac joint	60. Sacrum/coccyx
14. Gall bladder	30. Lymphatics	45. Leg	

Reflexology in the workplace, sport clubs, schools, hospices and hospitals

Reflexology is increasingly becoming integrated into the workplace, commercial companies and some hospitals and hospices are realising the benefits of reflexology for their staff as well as patients. VRT has a particular part to play in this field as the accelerated healing techniques mean that three people, instead of just one or two, can be treated in an hour with *complete VRT*. Complete VRT is a fully comprehensive reflexology treatment of 20–30 minutes which incorporates a few minutes of VRT techniques either side of conventional reflexology treatment (i.e before and after) and the deep relaxation of diaphragm rocking. Lynne Booth still recommends that a full 45- to 60-minute reflexology/VRT treatment is the preferred option, as the client is able to experience a longer period of rest and treatment. However, the accelerated response of VRT offers therapists an extremely useful tool to treat more people in a shorter space of time and is especially suitable for the elderly, chronically ill and young children. There is also a wide application for the use of VRT in the fields of sport, music, theatre, dance and commerce as well as in professions such as the police and fire service.

Conclusion

One of the reasons VRT has become well integrated into reflexology practice in the UK and internationally is that it is simple to learn and apply. Reflexology is a profound and non-invasive complementary therapy, and VRT is simply a unique and powerful skill to add to a therapist's repertoire.

Meridian therapy

Meridian therapy (or hand acupressure) is based on the theory of acupuncture and can be considered as acupuncture without needles. There are several different approaches which involve different theories, techniques, pressure and rhythms, and it can take years to master these techniques. In order to work effectively with meridian therapy it is essential to understand the paths of the meridians in the body and also to master one of the different acupuncture supporting frameworks such as Traditional Chinese Medicine, Yin and Yang theory, whether problems are due to deficiency or excess, and the Five Element theory.

Meridian system

An acupuncture meridian is an 'energy line' or 'energy pathway' inside the human body and is not that dissimilar to the ten longitudinal zones described in reflexology, but meridians are not as linear as those ten zones. Some reflexologists think that reflexology works through these meridians rather than the longitudinal zones, but neither theory has yet been proven.

There are 12 major meridians in the body, plus a few minor ones called extraordinary meridians, as well as some isolated points not linked to either major or minor meridians called extraordinary points. Most meridians run vertically, bilaterally and symmetrically. The 12 major meridians are named the lung, large intestine, stomach, spleen/pancreas, heart, small intestine, bladder, kidney, pericardium/circulation, triple burner, gall bladder and liver. Although the major meridians bear the names of organs of the body and they connect internally with those 12 organs, the theory behind their function is more complicated than just looking at Western diagnoses implicating these organs (e.g. a heart qi deficiency is not directly indicative of a heart disorder but involves the heart meridian and can be caused by a chronic illness).

The energy within a meridian is called *qi* or *chi* (pronounced 'chee') in Chinese medicine and is known as *Ki* in Japanese medicine. Qi is the life force or subtle energy that sustains all living things and it moves in one direction around the body. It travels throughout the whole body from the toes to the head and through the hands, and its main function is to transport qi and blood throughout the body. Illness results from an imbalance of this flow. Chinese medicine texts do not really describe disorders in terms of Western medicine as they are just manifestations that may or may not help with the diagnosis. Ten people with the same disorder, such as migraine, could have ten possible different diagnoses. Chinese medicine practitioners describe disharmonies in terms of the patterns that they manifest, and these are known as the Eight Fundamental Patterns or Eight Principles (interior, exterior, heat, cold, excess, deficiency, yin and yang).

Yin and yang

Meridians are classified as yin or yang on the basis of the direction in which the energy flows. Yin and yang are opposites, but harmony between these two elements means health, with yin seen as passive, female, interior and dark, and yang seen as active, male, exterior and light. Yin energy flows from the feet to the torso and from the torso along the inside of the arm to the fingertips. Yang energy flows from the fingertips to the face and along the back of the arm and from the face to the feet. There are approximately 340 or more acupuncture points over the whole body associated with the meridians. There are six meridians going through the arms and the hands: three yin (lung, pericardium and heart) and three yang (large intestine, sanjiao or triple warmer, and small intestine).

Five Element theory

The Five Element theory is used by some acupuncturists as a means of diagnosis and treatment. The five elements are wood, fire, earth, metal and water, and these can be related to body organs, body tissues, colours, seasons, directions, emotions and others. The relationship with body organs is that wood relates to the liver, fire to the heart, earth to the spleen/pancreas, metal to the lungs and water to the kidneys. An understanding of the elements helps to determine which organs and meridians are affected and which acupuncture points should be stimulated or sedated. The five elements show a law of cyclical interaction so, for example, fire can affect earth, earth affect metal, metal affect water, water affect wood and wood affect fire.

Positions of meridian points in the hands

For the six meridians that either begin (yang) or end (yin) in the fingers, the start/end positions are found just below the base of the nail and are as follows:

- Thumb – lung meridian (yin); a point on the outer side of the thumb just below the base of the nail. Problems associated with this meridian include pain, stiffness in the shoulder/elbow, carpal tunnel syndrome, tenosynovitis, arthritis in the thumb, warts and spots or ridges on the thumbnail.

- Index finger – large intestine meridian (yang); a point on the thumb side of the index finger just below the base of the nail. Problems associated with this meridian include nose bleeds, herpes on lips, throat problems, frozen shoulder, tennis elbow, greasy skin, as well as problems with the index finger and its nail.

- Middle finger – pericardium meridian (yin); a point on the index-finger side of the middle finger just below the base of the nail. Problems associated with this meridian include swollen axillary glands, carpal tunnel syndrome, hot palms, as well as problems with the middle finger and nail.

- Ring finger – triple warmer meridian (yang); a point on the little-finger side of the ring finger just below the base of the nail. Problems associated with this meridian include ear and eye problems, shoulder pains, stiffness and pain in the wrist and the arm, as well as problems with the ring finger (arthritis, eczema) or its nail.

- Little finger (palm) – heart meridian (yin); a point on the ring-finger side of the little finger just below the base of the nail. Problems associated with this meridian include speech defects, swollen axillary glands, inner arm problems, angina, weak wrists, stiffness, as well as problems with the little finger or its nail.

- Little finger (dorsum) – small intestine meridian (yang); a point on the inner side of the little finger just below the base of the nail. Problems associated with this meridian include tinnitus, deafness, trigeminal neuralgia, Bell's palsy, swollen glands in neck, aching and stiffness in the shoulder blade, tennis elbow, weak wrists, as well as problems with the little finger or white spots and ridging of its nail.

Techniques

Meridians are typically accessed through acupuncture points which act as 'gates' or 'entry points' as they are nearer the surface of the skin than the rest of the meridian to which they belong. Contact with these points can be made by using needles, burning an herb, using heat, tapping, using a blunt pointed instrument or simply pressing on the point.

The easiest technique to use is to apply firm pressure to the acupressure points being mindful of the type of pressure the client is used to or is able to stand. Apply pressure using either the thumbs, one of the other fingers (typically the index finger) or one of the knuckles (typically that of the index finger again) to apply stationary pressure. If an acupuncture point is very sensitive, you may gradually increase the pressure and hold without any movement for several minutes at a time. One minute of steady pressure, when applied gradually, calms and relaxes the nervous system. Other techniques may involve a rotating movement, either clockwise or anticlockwise, depending on whether you want to stimulate or sedate the point. Initially it is best to use firm pressure for one minute or more and see the effect it has on the client.

Some useful meridian points in the hands

With over 30 meridian points in the hands, those described below are a few which might be of particular use.

JOINING VALLEY

Joining Valley (Chinese name: Hegu; LI-4) is on the dorsal aspect of the hand, between the first and second metacarpal bones, at the midpoint of the second metacarpal bone and close to its radial border. Ask the client to squeeze their thumb against the tip of the index finger and locate LI-4 at the highest point of the bulge of the muscle and approximately level with the end of the crease. This point is often used for headaches, one-sided migraines or of the whole head,

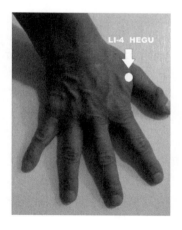

nasal congestion, tinnitus and allergies. It affects the whole face. It strengthens the body defensive qi, which is helpful for colds. Strong stimulation is contraindicated in pregnancy.

WRIST BONE

Wrist Bone (Chinese name: Wangu; SI-4) is on the ulnar border of the hand, in the depression between the base of the fifth metacarpal bone and the triquetral bone. This point is very useful for any wrist problems and used for neck, shoulder, cheek and submandibular region problems, and especially after whiplash. It is also used for tinnitus and in cases of jaundice. In cases of wrist issues, it works well with the Yang Valley point on the same meridian (the small intestine): the

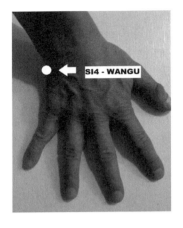

Yang Valley point (Yangu, SI-5), located at the ulnar border of the wrist, is in the depression between the head of the ulna and the triquetral bone.

SUPREME ABYSS

Supreme Abyss (Chinese name: Taiyuan; LU-9) is at the wrist joint, in the depression between the radial artery and the tendon of abductor pollicis longus. LU-9 tonifies the lung and promotes the downwards flow of qi from the lung. It can be used for a cough with watery phlegm, asthma, wheezing, dyspnoea and shortness of breath. This point is also used in cases of weakness or pain in the wrist, pain in the shoulder and back, pain in the supraclavicular fossa, pain in the medial aspect of the arm and breast pain.

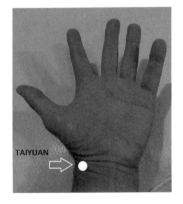

SPIRIT GATE

Spirit Gate (Chinese name: Shenmen; HE-7) is at the wrist joint, on the radial side of the flexor carpi ulnaris, in the depression at the proximal border of the pisiform bone. HE-7 calms the spirit as well as regulates and tonifies the heart. It is used for insomnia, frequent talking during sleep, poor memory, manic depression, epilepsy, dementia, heart pain and palpitations.

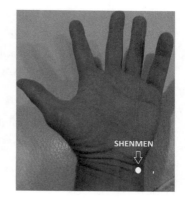

INNER PASS

Inner Pass (Chinese name: Neiguan; PC-6) is on the flexor aspect of the forearm, roughly two (thick) to three (thin) fingers breadth proximal to the crease of the wrist (approximately 3 cm) between the tendons of palmaris longus and flexor carpi radialis. PC-6 is very helpful to relieve nausea, especially if it is caused by sea or travel sickness or during pregnancy. This point regulates the heart, calms the spirit and harmonises the stomach.

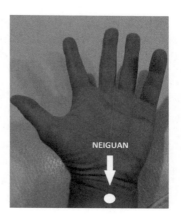

OUTER PASS

Outer Pass (Chinese name: Waiguan; SJ-5) is about 3 cm proximal to the dorsal wrist crease, in the depression between the radius and the ulna, on the radial side of the extensor digitorum communis tendons. SJ-5 benefits the head and the ears, helping with headaches (one-sided or frontal headaches) and dizziness. It also helps with constipation, abdominal pain as well as pain in the shoulder and back, stiff neck and numbness of the elbow.

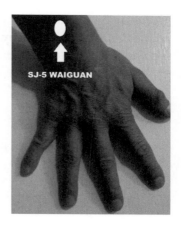

Points for tennis elbow

YANG STREAM

Yang Stream (Chinese name: Yangxi; LI-5) is on the radial side of the wrist, in the centre of the hollow formed by the tendons of extensor pollicis longus and brevis (the anatomical snuffbox).

VEERING PASSAGE

Veering Passage (Chinese name: Pianli; LI-6) is about 4 cm proximal to Yang Stream on the line connecting Yang Stream with Pool at the Crook (see next point).

POOL AT THE CROOK

Pool at the Crook (Chinese name: Quchi; LI-11) should be located with the elbow flexed and is located at the elbow, at the lateral end of the transverse cubital crease. LI-11 is also a powerful point for releasing stagnant qi in this region and relieves pain in the forearms, upper arm and shoulder. Pool at the Crook has several other 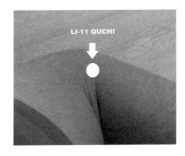 benefits: it is a powerful acupressure point to relieve constipation, digestive disorders, fever and inflammation. It is also used for skin conditions such as psoriasis and eczema.

Extraordinary points

There are 34 extraordinary points used in acupuncture. These points are not officially part of any meridians but are frequently used. One such point, Stiff Neck, is described below.

STIFF NECK

Stiff Neck (sometimes called Falling Down from Pillow; Chinese name: Luozhen) is on the dorsum of the hand between the second and third metacarpal bones, about 1–1.5 cm posterior to the metacarpophalangeal joint. This point is used for acute issues of the neck (i.e. strain, sprain and whiplash).

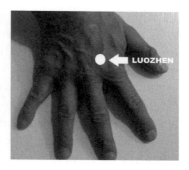

Chinese fingernail diagnosis

The practitioner of Traditional Chinese Medicine uses many methods of diagnosis, but one that may be of interest to practitioners of hand reflexology is that of fingernail diagnosis. The following different types of nail may indicate certain symptoms or deficiencies:

- Grooved nail: This may indicate a period of trauma or disease.

- Curved nail (curling down): This may indicate a cardiovascular disease or calcium deficiency.

- Concave nail (curling up): This may indicate a liver imbalance, arthritis or a spinal cord disease.

- Recessed grooves: This may indicate malnutrition, weak intestinal function or intestinal parasites.

- Short, wide nails: These may indicate a tendency towards disease affecting the abdomen, lumbar area and legs.

- Longitudinal striations: These may indicate malabsorption or deficiency of minerals.

Korean hand reflexology

Korean hand reflexology is a versatile and potent microsystem that was discovered by Dr Tae Woo Yoo. He once had a severe posterior headache, found a tender point on the back of the tip of his middle finger and was surprised to discover that the headache rapidly disappeared when he stimulated that point. He postulated that the middle finger of each hand represents the head. Between 1971 and

1975, Yoo extensively developed and studied the system and published his first textbook on this theory in 1977.

This new microsystem is simple to learn and safe to perform as it has minimal side effects. It offers mainly non-invasive treatment options with minimum pain or discomfort (pressure with a probe or use of acupressure discs) for maximum treatment effect. Therefore, the incidence of adverse events reported by the Korean Hand Therapy headquarters in Seoul is remarkably low (Yoo 2004).

In a clinical setting, Korean hand reflexology may combine with other treatments or therapies in four ways: effectively, simultaneously, alternatively and alternately (Dale 1990). It is also useful for people to learn simple treatment appropriate to them and use this to assist themselves between treatments at the clinic.

Possible mechanisms underlying Korean hand reflexology

The close link between the hands and the brain through the large territories associated with the hand in the motor cortex and sensory cortex of the brain suggests the important role of the hands in controlling all functions of the body. The stimulation of the hand points and areas, according to Korean hand reflexology theories, can modulate the autonomic nervous system by reducing or suppressing over-excited sympathetic nerves, thus restoring balance between the sympathetic and parasympathetic nervous systems. This is due to the presence of a large number of sympathetic nerve fibres condensely distributed on the hands with around the same amount as is found on the whole of the human body (Yoo 2009).

According to Korean hand reflexology theory, the left- and right-sided carotid and radial pulses should have a regular and equal blood flow, indicating a balanced flow to the brain and good circulation of blood and normal function of the internal organs. Korean hand reflexology treatment can control cerebral blood flow. Therefore, the purpose of treatment when the pulses are unbalanced is to regain normal balance throughout the body with the aim of improving health (Park and Yoo 2001).

Point locations on the hands

Korean hand reflexology theorises that the hands reflect the anatomy and physiology of the whole body. Furthermore, all the functions of the internal organs and tissues can be controlled by gentle stimulation of their corresponding points and areas on the hands for prevention, management and treatment of various diseases. Korean hand reflexology is theoretically unique and philosophically more profound than other microsystems. The aim of the treatment is to identify and stimulate the location of particular points or areas that correspond to that part of the body.

The palmar side represents the front of the body and the dorsal side represents the back of the body. The middle finger represents the head, neck and chest, the index and ring fingers represent the arms and the thumb and little fingers represent the legs.

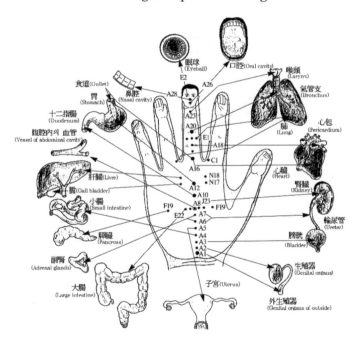

Korean hand reflexology: representation of the
body on the hand (palmar side)

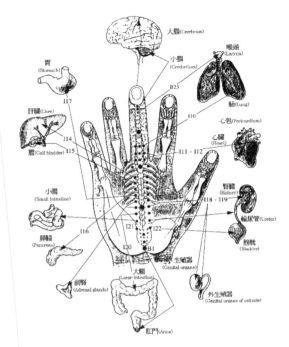

Korean hand reflexology: representation of the
body on the hand (dorsal side)

Treatment techniques in Korean hand reflexology

Dr Yoo developed a range of treatment techniques which vary
depending upon the onset, progress and conditions of both the patient
and the disease. Manual acupressure is the simplest and basic level of
treatment. Once the reactive corresponding point has been located,
acupressure can be applied to relieve or lessen the pain. Acupressure
can be applied either with the fingertip or using a therapeutic
instrument such as a probe; however, its effectiveness is limited to
cases of minor pain or symptoms which are in their early stages.

A more advanced level of treatment can be undertaken through
the application of acupressure discs. They are made of aluminium
and have one or numerous protrusions. The high conductivity of
aluminium acts to adjust the ionic imbalances in the body. Because
there is no involvement of skin penetration, acupressure discs can be
applied for a longer duration than manual acupressure thus extending

treatment effects. Application of acupressure discs can last from a few hours to a day; therefore, this method of treatment is particularly useful in long-term chronic illness or advanced symptoms.

Practical application of Korean hand reflexology

Korean hand reflexology treatments are very safe procedures and non-invasive; thus, the discomfort of treatment is minimised. It is an ideal treatment option for children, the elderly, the disabled and people who are nervous about invasive, painful treatments.

Several Korean hand reflexology studies published focus on paediatric (Jodorkovsky 1999), gynaecological and geriatric disorders. Results from a number of these studies suggest that Korean hand reflexology may be beneficial for menstrual symptoms (Lee and Choi 2005; Shin *et al.* 2004). It also may help reduce knee pain, shoulder pain and relieve constipation in elderly patients (An and Kim 2012; Kim, Kwon and Kim 2007; Lee and Kim 2010; Park *et al.* 2003).

Four studies have shown that the application of a capsicum plaster or capsaicin ointment on Korean hand reflexology point D2 reduced the incidence of postoperative nausea and vomiting (PONV) (Agarwal *et al.* 2005; Jung and Park 2013; Kim *et al.* 2002; Koo *et al.* 2013). Three studies have shown that the application of acupressure on Korean hand reflexology point K9 reduced the incidence of PONV and motion sickness (Bertalanffy *et al.* 2004; Boehler, Boehler and Puhringer 2002; Schlager, Mitterschiffthaler and Schlager 2000).

There have been some studies of the potential usefulness of Korean hand reflexology for certain illnesses; however, more extensive research into its use in the treatment of various health conditions is needed.

Conclusion

Korean hand reflexology is a theoretically unique and philosophically profound microsystem. Its well-defined theories and principles in diagnosis and treatments make it possible to perform the same potential functions as many other whole-body systems. It is useful to not only practitioners but also the general public since it is easy to learn, safe to use, cost-effective and practical to manage health and prevent diseases (Baik *et al.* 2014).

Chakras

Some approaches to reflexology treatment involve the chakras. The chakras are energy centres in the body through which energy flows. If there is a blockage in this energy flow, illness can result. There are seven major chakras positioned on the midline of the body from the base of the spine to the crown of the head, and each governs a specific function and can be linked to an endocrine gland. There are also 21 minor chakras. Each major chakra has its own vibrational frequency that is depicted through a specific chakra colour. The chakras can also be linked to reflexology reflex areas and, by working the appropriate reflex area in the hands, chakra-balancing can be achieved. The chakras can be identified in the hands in relation to the reflex area to the spine from the top of the thumb along the lateral border of the hand to the wrist.

Crown chakra

This is associated with the pineal gland and the colour violet. This chakra also works with the head.

Brow chakra

This is associated with the pituitary gland and the colour indigo. This chakra also works with the eyes, ears, nose mouth, back of head and forehead.

Throat chakra

This is associated with the thyroid and parathyroid glands and the colour blue. This chakra also works with the shoulders, arms and the hands.

Heart chakra

This is associated with the thymus and the colour green. This chakra also works with the heart, the breasts and the lungs.

Solar Plexus chakra

This is associated with the pancreas and the colour yellow. This chakra also works with the stomach, the spleen and the liver.

Sacral chakra

This is associated with the adrenals glands and the colour orange. This chakra relates to the female reproductive organs and the colon.

Base chakra

This is associated with the male reproductive glands and the colour red. This chakra also works with the legs, the feet and the scrotum.

Before working on the chakras in the hands, one must first determine whether or not each chakra is in balance and this is done through dowsing. If the chakra is out of balance it can be treated but if it is in balance then it should not be treated. Working the reflex areas in the hand is one approach to balancing the chakras; another approach is the use of colour and if a chakra is vibrating too fast then the complementary colour is used but if it is vibrating too slowly then the colour it vibrates to is used.

The chakras can be particularly helpful when there is hormonal imbalance in the body.

Hand and massage and aromatherapy

A full-body massage often includes massage to the hands, which in turn may include some specific massage to reflexology points. The same applies with aromatherapy massage when essential oils are used and absorbed into the skin with specific massage being given to specific points (usually acupressure) points to enhance the effectiveness. Even when having a manicure, hand massage is often offered to promote relaxation.

Care of the hands

There are other approaches to treatment involving the hands which may be of interest to the reflexologist, and just a few of those considered to be more significant are discussed in this book. With all the different points that can be found in the hands, the importance of the hands cannot be stressed enough. Care of the hands is important not just for their appearance through healthy-looking skin and nails but also for health. Damage to a part of the hand might affect the underlying reflex areas. By taking care of the hands you are taking care of the body since the whole body can be presented in the hands, so regular massage to the hands and precise massage using a method such as hand reflexology is very beneficial to health and well-being.

References

Agarwal, A., Dhiraaj, S., Tandon, M., Singh, P.K., Singh, U. and Pawar, S. (2005) 'Evaluation of capsaicin ointment at the Korean hand acupressure point K-D2 for prevention of postoperative nausea and vomiting.' *Anaesthesia 60*, 1185–1188.

An, Y.H. and Kim, Y.K. (2012) 'Effects of hands moxibustion therapy and hand press pellet on decreasing constipation among homebound elders.' *Korean Journal of Adult Nursing 2*, 24, 109–118.

Baik, J.K., Newman, I., Pokrysko, A., Heidelberger, E., Martindale, K. and Rooney, H. (2014) A Discussion of the Value of Korean Hand Therapy as a Preventative Medicine. *The 22nd Korea–Japan KHT Academic Seminar* book, pp.164–189. Seoul: Eumyangmekjin Publishing Co.

Bayly, D.E. (1988) *Reflexology Today*. Vermont: Healing Arts Press (original work published 1978).

Bertalanffy, P., Hoerauf, K., Fleischhackl, R., Strasser, H. *et al.* (2004) 'Korean hand acupressure for motion sickness in prehospital trauma care: a prospective, randomized, double-blinded trial in a geriatric population.' *Anesthesia & Analgesia 98*, 220–223.

Boehler, M., Mitterschiffthaler, G. and Schlager, A. (2002) 'Korean hand acupressure reduces postoperative nausea and vomiting after gynecological laparoscopic surgery.' *Anesthesia & Analgesia 94*, 872–875.

Carter, M. (1975) *Hand Reflexology: Key to Perfect Health*. New York: Parker Publishing Co Inc.

Dale, R.A. (1990) 'The Holograms of Hand Micro-Acupuncture: A Study in Systems of Correspondence.' *American Journal of Acupuncture 18*, 141–162.

Fitzgerald, W.H. and Bowers, E.F. (1980) *Zone Therapy*. California: Health Research (original work published 1917).

Ingham, E.D. and Byers, D. (1992) *The Original Works: Stories the Feet Can Tell Thru Reflexology and Stories the Feet Have Told Thru Reflexology*. Florida: Ingham Publishing Inc (original works published 1938 and 1959).

Jodorkovsky, R. (1999) 'Hand acupuncture experience in pediatric patients.' *Medical Acupuncture 11*, 25–28.

Jung, H.J. and Park, S.Y. (2013) 'Combination of capsicum plaster at the Korean hand acupuncture points K-D2 with prophylactic antiemetic on postoperative nausea and vomiting after gynecologic laparoscopy.' *Journal of the Korean Academy of Nursing 43*, 215–224.

Kim, K.S., Koo, M.S., Jeon, J.W., Park, H.S. and Seung, I.S. (2002) 'Capsicum plaster at the Korean hand acupuncture point reduces postoperative nausea and vomiting after abdominal hysterectomy.' *Anesthesia & Analgesia 95*, 1103–1107.

Kim, N.J., Kwon, Y.S. and Kim, H.D. (2007) 'The effects of Koryo hand moxibustion therapy on the constipation of old adults in community.' *Journal of Korean Clinical Nursing Research 13*, 37–49.

Koo, M.S., Kim, K.S., Lee, H.J., Jeong, J.S. and Lee, J.W. (2013) 'Antiemetic efficacy of capsicum plaster on acupuncture points in patients undergoing thyroid operation.' *Korean Journal of Anesthesiology 65*, 539–543.

Lee, I.S. and Choi, H.S. (2005) 'Effect of self moxibustion on dysmenorrhea and activities of daily living in female college students.' *Korean Journal of Women Health Nursing 11*, 1, 77–82.

Lee, Y.O. and Kim, C.N. (2010) 'The effects of hand acupuncture: Moxibustion therapy on elders' shoulder pain, ADL/IADL and sleep disorders.' *Journal of the Korean Academy of Community Health Nursing 21*, 229–241.

Park, J.S., Woo, S.N., Yeo, H.J. and Kim, K.S. (2003) 'The effect of hand moxibustion therapy on knee joint pain, joint range of motion and discomfort during ADL in elderly people.' *Journal of Korean Academy of Fundamental Nursing 10*, 244–253.

Park, K.H. and Yoo, T.W. (2001) 'The change of cerebral blood flow before and after treatment of Koryo hand therapy.' *The Internet Journal of Alternative Medicine 2001*, 1, 1.

Riley, J.S. (2010) *Zone Therapy Simplified*. Montana: Kessinger Publishing, LLC (original work published 1919).

Schlager, A., Boehler, M. and Puhringer, F. (2000) 'Korean hand acupressure reduces postoperative vomiting in children after strabismus surgery.' *British Journal of Anaesthesia 85*, 267–270.

Shin, K.-R., Kim, K.-H., Kim, H.-S., Kim, E.-H., Lee, J.-R. and Kim, J.-H. (2004) 'The effect of hand moxibustion therapy on pain during menstruation.' *Korean Journal of Adult Nursing 16*, 256–263.

Yoo, T.W. (2004) *Koryo Soojichim Gangjwa* [The Lecture on Korean Hand Acupuncture] (volume 1) (pp.230–238). Seoul: Eumyangmekjin Publishing Co.

Yoo, T.W. (2009) *Koryo Soojichim Gangjwa* [The Lecture on Korean Hand Acupuncture]. Seoul: Koryo Soojichim.

Resources

THE BAYLY SCHOOL OF REFLEXOLOGY

Nicola Hall is director of the Bayly School of Reflexology, the official teaching body of the British Reflexology Association. The Bayly School was established in 1979 and has trained many thousands of reflexology practitioners around the world with courses in London, Birmingham, Worcester, Scotland, Switzerland, Kenya and Japan.

Monks Orchard, Whitbourne, Worcester WR6 5RB
Tel: (+44) (0)1886 821207
E-mail: bayly@britreflex.co.uk
Website: www.britreflex.co.uk

LYNNE BOOTH (VERTICAL HAND REFLEXOLOGY)
BA HONS, BRCP, IIR, ART HONS, HMAR HONS, FHT

Lynne began studying reflexology 25 years ago and went on to train with the International Institute of Reflexology (original Ingham method). She has a private practice and also runs a reflexology clinic at a 400-resident St Monica Trust in Bristol as well as a clinic for professional championship footballers. The research, development of VRT and the small medical study were conducted at the Trust in the early to mid-1990s. She frequently presents VRT at conferences internationally. She is the author of *Vertical Reflexology* published by Piatkus Books in September 2000 and *Vertical Reflexology for Hands*, published in 2002. She has also produced a VRT dvd and VRT hand and foot dorsal charts.

Booth VRT Ltd
Suite 205, 60 Westbury Hill, Bristol BS9 3UJ
Tel: (+44) (0)1179 626746
E-mail: contact@boothvrt.com
Website: www.boothvrt.com

PHILIPPE MATHON (ACUPUNCTURIST)

Philippe trained at The London College of Traditional Acupuncture and Chinese Medicine in 2000. He is qualified in acupuncture (Traditional Chinese Medicine and Japanese), massage, shiatsu, hypnotherapy and is a yoga teacher. He is also a reflexologist having trained with the Bayly School of Reflexology in 2000.

406 Edgware Road, London W2 1ED
Tel: (+44) (0)20 3674 0855
E-mail: emails@philippemathon.com
Website: www.PhilippeMathon.com

JONG BAIK (KOREAN HAND REFLEXOLOGY)

Jong Baik is an acupuncturist and lecturer who originally studied Korean hand therapy in South Korea in the early 1990s. He runs a clinic in Darlington, County Durham, specialising in palliative care. He also travels the world lecturing on microsystems and Traditional East Asian Medicine. For more information about Jong and opportunities to learn more about Korean hand therapy, please visit his website.

Tel: (+44) (0)1325 367179
E-mail: info@JongBaik.co.uk
Website: www.JongBaik.co.uk

THE BRITISH REFLEXOLOGY ASSOCIATION (BRA)

The BRA was founded in 1985 as a representative body for reflexology practitioners trained in the Bayly method.

Administration Office, Monks Orchard,
Whitbourne, Worcester WR6 5RB
Tel: (+44) (0)1886 821207
E-mail: bra@britreflex.co.uk
Website: www.britreflex.co.uk

COMPLEMENTARY AND NATURAL HEALTHCARE COUNCIL (CNHC)

The CNHC was set up with government support in 2008 to protect the public by providing a UK voluntary register of complementary therapists. The CNHC's register has been approved as an Accredited Register by the Professional Standards Authority for Health and Social Care.

Tel: (+44) (0)207 653 1971
E-mail: info@cnhc.org.uk
Website: www.cnhc.org.uk

INTEGRATED HEALTHCARE PARTNERSHIP LIMITED

The Integrated Healthcare Partnership is a specialist healthcare consultancy, online iCAMhub and community wellness scheme which works to support the development of integrated healthcare across the UK. The iCAMhub is the one-stop resource for finding and rating a practitioner or service in the UK.

Suite 150, 34 Buckingham Palace Road, London SW1W 0RH
Tel: (+44) (0)7970 052978
E-mail: office@iCAMhub.com
Website: www.iCAMhub.com or
www.integratedhealthcarepartnership.com

Index

skin 45, 105, 115, 121, 138, 144, 146,
147, 148–9, 165, 169, 174, 181, 196
see also integumentary system
small intestine 40–1, 68, 91, 140, 145,
146, 190, 191, 192, 194
solar plexus 38, 66, 80, 90, 104, 107, 176,
178, 202
spine 51, 59, 82, 108, 111, 114, 136, 138,
162, 164, 177, 178, 202
spleen 31, 38, 39, 90, 165, 169, 176, 190,
191, 202
sternum 46, 47, 108
stomach 38, 39–40, 68, 91, 140, 141,
168, 190, 195, 202
stomach ulcer 144
stress 14, 42, 107, 116, 123, 136, 139,
141, 146, 149, 154, 163, 164, 176,
178
stroke 134, 139, 140, 162

teeth 43, 45, 61, 84, 140
tendonitis 114
testis 48, 49, 50, 75, 99, 115, 127–8
throat 36, 45, 159, 192, 202
thrush 127, 169–70
thymus 36, 38, 165, 202
thyroid 34, 36, 37, 65, 88, 115, 120–1,
123, 125, 151, 164, 172, 177, 202
tinnitus 105, 133, 163, 192, 193, 194
toothache 140, 177

ureter tube 40, 42, 71, 94, 149, 175
urethritis 151
urinary system 105, 149
disorders 149–51
reflex areas 152–3
uterus 48, 49, 50, 76, 100, 115, 122,
124–5, 127, 151, 175

vaginitis 127
varicose veins 145, 164
vas deferens 48, 50, 76, 99, 115, 127
vertical reflex therapy (VRT) 183–9
vertigo 134

wrist 22, 25, 28, 29, 47, 64, 87, 79, 103,
108, 186, 194
problems 112, 114, 115, 169, 180, 181,
192

zone related areas (cross reflexes) 22
zone therapy 16–17
zones
longitudinal 16–17, 21–2, 34, 190
transverse 19–21, 32, 51